CONTENTS

Cover design by Harby Bonello.

ISBN 9780965877794 $29.95 US/CAN

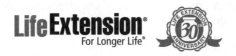

1100 W. Commercial Blvd. Fort Lauderdale, FL 33309
1-800-544-4440 • www.lef.org

FOREWORD

There are so many misconceptions about why aging people gain unwanted fat pounds that this book simply had to be written.

Americans live in an egregious state of denial concerning their metabolic capacity to process the excess calories they ingest each day. What people fail to grasp is that as their bodies age, they are no longer able to handle the calorie burden the same way they did in their youth.

The combination of excess calories and age-related metabolic changes conspires to produce unsightly body fat. Furthermore, when fat stores accumulate around our internal organs in the abdominal region (visceral fat), risks for age-related diseases like heart attack and stroke increase sharply.

While type II diabetes and cardiovascular disease are the disorders most frequently associated with abdominal obesity, a plethora of research links a diverse number of lethal illnesses to the bulge in our bellies.

This book does far more than provide a comprehensive, integrated program to enable you to lose weight. By following these weight loss protocols, you will simultaneously protect against the most common medical problems aging individuals face.

Perhaps the most graphic way to emphasize the deleterious impact of ingested calories is for you to take an FDA-approved drug called *orlistat* (available over-the-counter under the brand name alli®). You will soon observe gobs of fat floating in your feces that this drug inhibited you from absorbing.

What should shock you most is that orlistat, at a dose of 120 mg taken three times a day, only impeded the absorption of about **30%** of those fat calories. The remaining **70%** of the dietary fats you ate are circulating in your bloodstream, or have been stored by your already bloated adipocytes (fat cells).

The **Life Extension Weight Loss Guide** identifies a wide range of proven obesity-inducers and, most importantly, provides practical steps that can enable you to circumvent each and every one of them.

Recommendations in this book are supported by findings from the peer-reviewed scientific literature. Yet no one has yet tied these discoveries together into a cohesive program to combat the multiple factors that underlie age-associated weight gain.

For instance, there is a generic drug called *acarbose* that inhibits carbohydrate digestive enzymes like *alpha-glucosidase*, *maltase*, and *sucrase*. This medication reliably reduces post-meal blood sugar levels by about 20% after a high-carbohydrate meal. It also helps reduce the dangerous surge of insulin release associated with high-carbohydrate meals. Yet because this drug long ago came off patent for treatment of type 2 diabetes, pharmaceutical companies don't promote it and most physicians have forgotten it. The good news for those seeking to slow their *absorption* of carbohydrates is that acarbose is widely available as a low-cost generic. By itself, acarbose will not induce significant weight loss. When combined with the other fat-loss modalities described in this book, however, acarbose adds a unique weapon to enable you to restore your metabolic capacity to shed excess fat pounds.

The **Life Extension Weight Loss Guide** will forever change your perceptions about why people gain weight as they age and how critically important it is to follow a comprehensive program to achieve significant and sustained fat loss.

— William Faloon
Co-Founder, Life Extension

PREFACE

Why do we find it so hard to shed surplus fat pounds?

As you are about to learn, too many have become <u>addicted</u> to a lifestyle that virtually guarantees chronic age-associated weight gain, especially in the **abdominal** region.

The good news is that when properly utilized in combination with a reduced-calorie diet and exercise, currently available nutrients, drugs, and hormones can thwart these insidious **obesity-inducers.** In fact, the underlying scientific data supporting these approaches are quite impressive. But what was lacking until now is a cohesive approach incorporating <u>all</u> of these discoveries into a comprehensive weight-loss program.

For example, drugs that <u>block</u> dietary **fat** *absorption* into the bloodstream have **proven** efficacy.[6-9] Using this fat-blocking method alone, however, fails to meet the expectations of most overweight individuals. One reason is that excess **carbohydrate absorption** will cause the same disruption of **metabolic processes** as overconsumption of **dietary fats.**

On the flip side, drugs or nutrients that block the rate of **carbohydrate** <u>absorption</u> may not induce profound weight loss if too many **dietary fats** wind up in the bloodstream.

What people fail to accept is that as they grow older, they lack the **metabolic capacity** to efficiently convert ingested calories into energy. These metabolic <u>deficits</u> are increasingly being referred to as "postprandial disorders." The term *postprandial* means **after-meal**, and the <u>disorders</u> they refer to are <u>too</u> many **fats** and **sugars** remaining in the bloodstream long after meals are eaten.

Overweight individuals today suffer chronically high blood levels of fat remnants and glucose that may frustrate the best laid-out weight-loss program.[8,10]

One might think that by merely eating less, blood fat (triglycerides) and sugar (glucose) levels will drop low enough to prompt weight reduction. The harsh reality is that many overweight individuals are so severely compromised on a metabolic and hormonal basis that sustained fat loss *cannot* be achieved unless corrective actions are first taken. An imbalance of leptin, insulin, thyroid, and/or sex steroid hormones, for example, may inhibit the desired release of stored body fat, even in response to calorie restriction.

As humans age, there is a progressive and extensive decline in *resting energy expenditure*. This reduction in **basal metabolic rate** is another reason that people accumulate more body fat even though they may be eating less than they used to. In fact, your body's basal metabolic rate decreases by about 2% per decade after age 40. For a man who is 40 years old and weighs 156 pounds this means that during the year following his 50th birthday, he is predisposed to gain an extra **3.5 pounds of body fat** from the age-related reduction in metabolic rate *alone* compared with his metabolic rate at age 40![98] Metabolic enhancers by themselves, however, are not enough to compensate for the *other* obesity-inducers plaguing aging adults.

In response to compelling evidence that unwanted weight gain is a multi-factorial process, Life Extension® has developed the comprehensive fat-loss program you are about to read. *The Life Extension Weight Loss Guide* is a culmination of over 30 years of investigation into the multiple causes of age-related weight gain and what can be done to reverse these deadly processes.

CHAPTER 1

Nine Pillars of Successful Weight Loss

When it comes to *weight loss,* mainstream medicine has recommended "diet and exercise" for so long, it has become more of a cliché than a momentous scientific communication.

The fact is that as people get older, they need to do a lot <u>more</u> than reduce calorie intake and increase physical activity to lose excess body fat and keep it off.

In this chapter, we address the <u>nine</u> steps that most overweight aging people should follow to achieve optimal removal of surplus body fat. This multi-step program is comparable to the "drug cocktails" doctors now use to control HIV infections (so patients now live for decades instead of less than a year, as was the case when the disease first manifested).

The *Nine Pillars of Successful Weight Loss* are also analogous to what progressive oncologists are doing to cure cancer today by administering multiple therapies designed to neutralize the numerous survival mechanisms cancer cells use to escape eradication.

In some respects, the uncontrolled proliferation and enlargement of adipocytes (fat cells) in the aging body is analogous to the growth and spread of benign tumors in our abdomens, buttocks, and other areas of the body.

Most people understand the need to correct vascular disease risk factors (such as elevated LDL, triglycerides and C-reactive protein) to protect against heart attack and stroke. In the same way, those seeking to lose weight should make many of these *Nine Pillars of Successful Weight Loss* a regular part of their health-maintenance program to not only shed body fat, but also slash cardiovascular, diabetes and cancer risks.

Pillar Number 1:
Restore Insulin Sensitivity

Normal aging causes a decline in sex hormones and anabolic hormone production. In addition, insulin receptors on cell membranes lose their youthful sensitivity or functionality. The result is a

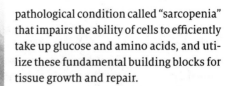

pathological condition called "sarcopenia" that impairs the ability of cells to efficiently take up glucose and amino acids, and utilize these fundamental building blocks for tissue growth and repair.

"Insulin resistance" is characterized by the relative difficulty of muscle cells and liver cells to take up glucose. Hyperinsulinemia, a condition of high circulating insulin levels, is the body's response to insulin resistance (the attempt to produce more insulin to "drive" more glucose into cells). However, an increased risk of heart disease is well-known to be associated with high circulating insulin levels. In fact, a recent study showed that patients with heart disease had significantly higher plasma levels of blood sugar and circulating insulin.[17]

There are several ways to restore insulin sensitivity to our cell membranes. For example, nutrients such as *chromium*,[18,19] *magnesium*,[20] *and fish oil* [21,22] can help.

A low-cost prescription drug called *metformin* can also significantly enhance insulin sensitivity.[23-25] It is approved only as a treatment for type 2 diabetes, but published scientific studies indicate it can help improve metabolic function, reduce food intake, and lower body fat in obese, non-diabetic individuals.[26] The dose range for metformin in those individuals without type 2 diabetes seeking to enhance their insulin sensitivity and support more youthful metabolic function is usually 500–1,000 mg daily, but individual needs & tolerability vary. Consult with your prescribing physician to make sure that metformin is right for you. As you will read later in this section, restoring free *testosterone* to youthful ranges can also augment insulin sensitivity in aging men with suboptimal testosterone levels.

The most effective way of restoring insulin sensitivity is to reduce calorie intake. Calorie reduction to 1,500–1,900 calories/day significantly enhances insulin sensitivity, as documented by dramatic lowering of fasting glucose and insulin blood levels.[26-31] Even a moderate cutback of excess calories can markedly improve insulin sensitivity.

So the first pillar to successful long-term weight loss should involve a moderate reduction in calorie intake, at least long enough to restore insulin receptor sensitivity to more youthful ranges. The use of nutrients, hormones, and medications that enhance insulin sensitivity should also be considered. As you probably already know, you need to do a lot more than just eat less to lose weight.

Pillar Number 2:
Restore Youthful Hormone Balance

Most overweight people have suffered the agonies of calorie deprivation (dieting) but have failed to achieve any kind of sustained fat reduction. While eating less addresses some of the underlying causes of weight gain, the high failure rate of dieting is partially attributable to the severe alteration in *hormone* levels that occurs as part of normal aging.

A large percentage of men today suffer from abdominal obesity, the most dangerous kind of body fat. It is often difficult, if not impossible, for aging men to lose inches off their waistlines if they are deficient in *free testosterone,* especially in the presence of *excess estrogen.*[32-34] Low levels of *dehydroepiandrosterone* (DHEA) can also contribute to undesirable fat accumulation in men and women.[35]

A comprehensive blood test panel can reveal free testosterone and estrogen (estradiol) levels so that a physician can prescribe a topical testosterone cream and an *aromatase-inhibiting* drug (if necessary) to restore a man's sex hormone profile to a youthful range. The same blood test panel can also detect DHEA blood levels to enable one to take the proper dose of this over-the-counter dietary supplement.

A comprehensive blood test panel should also measure prostate-specific antigen (PSA) in men (along with a digital rectal exam, and prostate ultrasound with biopsy, if necessary) to help screen for occult prostate cancer. Those with prostate cancer usually cannot restore these hormones until the cancer is eradicated. Some men are able to reduce excess estrogen and simultaneously boost free testosterone by taking nutrient formulas that contain plant extracts to help inhibit the aromatase enzyme (which converts testosterone into estrogen) and decrease levels of *sex hormone-binding globulin* (which binds free testosterone).

A substantial percentage of aging women (and many aging men) have less-than-optimal thyroid levels due to a sluggish thyroid, a condition known as hypothyroidism, which predisposes them to weight gain. Thyroid hormone is needed to maintain healthy metabolic rates. Those who suffer from a deficiency in thyroid hormone should be prescribed thyroid medication. Medications to consider are *Armour® natural thyroid complex* (containing both T4 and T3) or Cytomel® (containing T3). Trying to lose weight in the face of thyroid hormone deficit can be particularly challenging.

A common problem women experience during menopause is an *increase* in belly fat mass. Estrogen levels plummet during menopause and some studies correlate this *estrogen deficiency* with greater abdominal adiposity in women. While treatment with high dosages of horse urine-derived estrogens and pro-gestin drugs may contribute to increases in appetite and weight gain, evidence suggests that individually dosed natural estrogen replacement facilitates a reduction in abdominal fat in women who are estrogen deficient.[36,37] Restoring hormone balance in aging females requires the intervention of a health care prac-titioner with specialized expertise in prescribing *bioidentical hormone replacement therapy.* Men are more fortunate in that almost any doctor can prescribe the proper dose of testosterone (and aromatase-inhibiting drugs, if needed).

Pillar Number 3:
Control Rate of Carbohydrate Absorption

In response to eating a large meal, people gain fat pounds because of the rapid rise in blood glucose (and the subsequent insulin spike). Large meals first overload the bloodstream with calories and later cause a rebound increase in appetite when blood sugar levels plummet in response to excess release of insulin. Research suggests that by taking just five grams of soluble fiber before or with each meal, one can significantly blunt the glucose-insulin surge.[38]

Fiber may protect against unwanted weight gain via several mechanisms that involve both effects on satiety and glucose-insu-lin responses.[38-40] For example, research has shown that vegetarians weigh significantly less than non-vegetarians, whether measured by body mass index or body weight.[41] Some experts believe that vegetarians' lower average body weight is linked to one factor: the high fiber content of the plant foods consumed.[42] Plant fiber fills you up quickly, and studies indicate that this results in less snacking and binging later in the day.

The *Seven Countries Study* provides additional evidence linking a high-fiber diet with lower body weight. Researchers found that people living in countries with high fiber intake weighed less than those living in countries where fiber intake is low.[43] Higher fiber intake is also associated with lower average body weight in the US. In the famous *Nurses' Health Study,* those who ingested more dietary fiber consistently weighed less than those who consumed less fiber.[40]

Finally, in the *Coronary Artery Risk Development in Young Adults Study*, which examined how heart disease develops in adults, researchers linked higher dietary fiber intake with lower body weight and waist-to-hip ratios, along with a reduction in markers of heart disease risk. Higher fiber consumption predicted less weight gain more strongly than did total or saturated fat consumption.[42]

Not all fibers are created equal. Beta-glucans (derived from oats and barley) are particularly effective in slowing the absorption of carbohydrates — enabling one to control blood sugar levels and induce the satiety needed to achieve healthy weight management. Studies show that when taken with meals, beta-glucan fibers markedly blunt post-meal elevations in blood sugar and insulin levels. Like other foods rich in soluble fiber, beta-glucans help improve blood glucose metabolism while also lowering serum lipid levels.[44,45]

Getting into the routine of taking five grams of a neutral-tasting beta-glucan fiber mix before or with each meal would help provide weight loss effects via this mechanism (i.e., controlling rate of carbohydrate absorption). Alternatively, taking fiber capsules (containing the highly viscous fiber glucomannan, which promotes healthy glycemic status) before each carbohydrate-rich meal would also help reduce the glucose-insulin surge that contributes to obesity.

Some people with chronic weight control problems will need more than soluble fibers to delay the rapid rise in blood sugar and insulin in association with dietary carbohydrate *consumption. Excess ingestion of fiber-poor carbohydrates* in our diet, like sugar and white flour, contribute to surplus body fat by rapidly increasing blood sugar and by converting to *triglycerides* that bloat our fat cells. Compounds that slow the rate of complex and simple carbohydrate breakdown and absorption can be important components of a weight management program.

Alpha-glucosidase is an enzyme that helps with the breakdown of simple carbohydrates into glucose. *Alpha-amylase is an enzyme that* helps with the breakdown of large carbohydrate molecules like starch into glucose polymers (linked chains of glucose molecules). These simple sugars are then broken down to glucose by the *alpha-glucosidase* enzyme. Pharmaceutical agents known to target *alpha-amylase* and *alpha-glucosidase* include the drug *acarbose*, with the end result being a less rapid rise in blood sugar and insulin levels in response to carbohydrate ingestion. Extracts of some specific nutrients have also been shown to target these enzymes.

For example, an extract from the white kidney bean *(Phaseolus vulgaris)* targets the *alpha-amylase enzyme and helps reduce the rapid increase in blood glucose after consumption of a carbohydrate-rich meal.* In a placebo-controlled study, those taking white kidney bean extract before meals lost **1.5 inches** of **abdominal fat** over an 8-week period.

Another example is *L-arabinose*, a natural substance found in certain plants. *L-arabinose* targets the *sucrase* enzyme, helping to delay the rapid rise in blood sugar associated with sucrose consumption. Americans eat far too much sucrose. In fact, a USDA study in 1999 showed that Americans consumed an average of <u>158 pounds of sucrose per person</u>, and that this was *30% higher* than in 1983![46]

Experimental studies show that when animals are fed sucrose, *L-arabinose* helps significantly reduce the amount of sugar converted into fat in the animals' liver.[47]

Furthermore, a 28-day human clinical study shows that a combination of *L-arabinose* and chromium can help reduce the rapid increase in blood sugar in response to consumption of sucrose by an average of 25%.[48]

Medications and nutrients shown to be effective in blunting the sharp glucose/insulin surge in response to ingestion of dietary carbohydrates include:

Beta-glucan (soluble fiber powder)	5–10 grams
Acarbose (generic prescription drug)	50–100 mg
Metformin (generic prescription drug)	250–850 mg
Phase 3™ (*L-arabinose*)	550 mg
Phase 2™ (white kidney bean extact)	445 mg

The above nutrients and drugs should be taken <u>before</u> meals for optimal results.

Pillar Number 4:
Increase Physical Activity

Most people think the only weight-loss benefit of exercise is to use up more stored body fat calories. In reality, exercise induces many beneficial changes at the cellular level that contribute to better weight control. Increased physical activity itself improves insulin sensitivity and mimics the effect of certain anti-diabetic drugs (such as the PPAR-gamma agonists), which can have a favorable effect on body fat distribution.[59]

The type and intensity of physical activity will vary considerably among individuals. The reason *increased physical activity* is one of the *Nine Pillars of Successful Weight Loss* is to encourage everyone seeking optimal fat loss to engage in some form of increased physical activity. Even a modest increase in physical activity should produce some reduction of fat mass (especially in the abdomen) enough to motivate even sedentary individuals to become more consistently physically active.

(Continued on page 16) 13

Where's the Fat?

The location of body fat stores is directly related to disease risk factors. People with excess levels of abdominal fat are at markedly increased risk of chronic illnesses such as cardiovascular disease and type 2 diabetes — both of which are closely related to the metabolic syndrome.[49,50] Direct entry of fats from abdominal stores into the liver may trigger increased insulin resistance, accounting for the relationship with type 2 diabetes.[51]

Recent studies have also shown that the potent endocrine function of abdominal body fat may explain the relationship between abdominal fat and cognitive decline, such as that seen in Alzheimer's and other neurodegenerative diseases.[52]

Abdominal fat is not just a problem in adults. New studies have established a relationship between fat distribution in early childhood and adolescence and serious chronic disease in early to mid-adulthood.[53,54] Responsible doctors now include abdominal circumference measurements at routine visits as a means of identifying these risk factors.[55]

Even within the abdomen, the location of fat stores matters. People with excessive amounts of fat in their livers (fatty liver disease) are at even higher risk for all of these chronic conditions, compared with those who have lower levels of liver fat.[56] Indeed, damage to liver cells, as measured by increased levels of liver-based enzymes in the bloodstream, is closely associated with decreased insulin sensitivity and is a risk factor for development of type 2 diabetes.[57,58]

Fat and Oxidative Stress

Because of its chemical nature, fat is readily oxidized by free radicals — and it is the oxidized form of many lipids that triggers the blood vessel damage and eventual plaque formation that leads to atherosclerosis. Obesity is closely associated with increased oxidative stress,[66] while loss of body fat is associated with decreasing levels of molecules associated with oxidation.[67] The bottom line is that people with excessive adipose tissue are walking "oxidant factories" whose bodies must cope with enormous loads of these violently destructive molecules.

Fat and Inflammation

The metabolic syndrome and its related conditions all derive from increased levels of inflammatory molecules called cytokines — more prominently found in people with excessive stores of body fat.[50,68] Indeed, physicians now commonly measure certain markers of inflammation such as C-reactive protein (CRP) as a means of screening for people at risk for cardiovascular disease.[69] Fortunately, reductions in body fat content (through exercise, diet, and appropriate supplementation) are associated with healthy reductions in inflammatory markers — and that means a reduction in the many risk factors associated with obesity-related inflammation.[70-72]

Fat and Cancer

Excess body fat not only increases the risk of cardiovascular disease, it also increases the risk of deadly cancers. In one large European study, increasing body mass index was associated with a significant increase in the risk of cancer for 10 out of 17 specific types examined.[80] Recent studies have shown a powerful association between body fat content and kidney and liver cancers.[81,82] By now, it should be no surprise that weight loss, specifically body fat reduction, can lead to lowered risks for cancers.[83,84] One study has estimated a reduction of 45% in the risk of breast cancer in women who lost more than about nine pounds.[84]

Fat and Cardiovascular Disease

High body fat is strongly associated with cardiovascular disease. But the relationship is more complicated and subtle than we thought. Atherosclerosis is the result of the cycle of lipid oxidation, inflammation, and vascular injury. But fat tissue causes other risks independent of plasma lipid levels. Acting as an endocrine organ, fat tissue can increase the flow of hormones (adipokines) involved in blood pressure control.[51,86] It seems to be the accumulation of abdominal fat that produces these remarkable and deadly effects.[87] It is fortunate that adequate reduction in body fat content through lifestyle changes, diet, and supplementation has been associated with decreased risk for cardiovascular catastrophes like heart attacks and strokes.[88-91]

Controlling Body Fat Content Safely

Despite the obvious dangers of obesity, specifically elevated abdominal body fat content, most Americans have a hard time losing weight. Many turn to drastic solutions such as bariatric surgery ("stomach stapling"), which does provide some benefit in extreme cases,[94] or to "diet pills" that often contain dangerous central nervous system (CNS) stimulants.[95-99]

Pillar Number 5:
Restore Brain Serotonin

When the brain is flooded with serotonin, satiety normally occurs. A serotonin deficiency has been associated with the *carbohydrate binging* that contributes to the accumulation of excess body fat.[60] Some studies suggest that obese individuals have a tendency towards low blood tryptophan levels, which suggests that their overeating patterns may be related to a serotonin deficiency in the brain.[61,62]

In addition, cutting-edge research reveals that chronic inflammation and immune system overactivation appear to play critical roles in obesity.[62,63] Inflammatory cytokines like interferon-gamma are made and released in body fat. An enzyme called *indoleamine 2,3-dioxygenase* is activated by interferon-gamma, which then *degrades* tryptophan in the body. *Tryptophan is needed* to produce *serotonin* in the brain.

Furthermore, human studies suggest that obese patients have *decreased* plasma tryptophan levels that remain low, *independent* of weight reduction or dietary intake.[61,62] This altered **tryptophan** metabolism reduces **serotonin** production and contributes to impaired satiety, which in turn contributes to increased caloric intake and obesity.

When obese patients were given 1,000 mg, 2,000 mg, or 3,000 mg doses of L-tryptophan one hour before meals, a significant *decrease* in caloric consumption was observed. The majority of the reduction in caloric intake was in the amount of *carbohydrates* consumed and not the amount of protein consumed.[64]

In a double-blind, placebo-controlled study, obese patients on protein-rich diets who received tryptophan (750 mg, twice daily, orally) experienced significant weight loss, compared with a placebo group.[65]

Those seeking to embark on a *comprehensive* weight-loss program should consider adding *tryptophan* (along with nutrients that inhibit tryptophan-degrading enzymes) to their daily program in starting doses of 500 mg before meals, two to three times per day.

Pillar Number 6:
Restore Resting Energy Expenditure Rate

It is often hard to lose significant body fat stores even when following a low-calorie diet, restoring youthful hormone balance, ingesting fiber, and aggressively exercising. A missing link is boosting *resting energy expenditure,* i.e., **burning off stored body fat.**

Several natural nutritional agents offer safe and effective means of enhancing metabolic rate without stimulating the central nervous system (CNS) and causing unsafe increases in blood pressure such as with Ma Huang and/ or ephedrine. They include:

• **The green tea polyphenol, epigallocatechin gallate (EGCG)**. In combination with caffeine (50 mg caffeine, 90 mg EGCG) EGCG has been shown to enhance 24-hour energy expenditure in human test subjects. In this same clinical study, treatment with caffeine alone had no effect upon energy expenditure, indicating that the effect of green tea in promoting fat burning goes beyond its caffeine content.[73] Other scientific data indicate that green tea polyphenols in combination with caffeine synergistically enhance thermogenesis (fat burning).[74]

• **Fish oils rich in EPA and DHA**. Although many people are aware of the cardiovascular benefits of fish oils rich in EPA and DHA, few people know that these omega-3 fatty acids have beneficial effects on thermogenesis. They inhibit key enzymes responsible for lipid synthesis, such as fatty acid synthase and stearoyl-CoA desaturase-1, enhance lipid oxidation and fat burning, and inhibit free fatty acids from entering adipocytes (fat cells) for fat storage.[75]

• **Conjugated linoleic acid**. Experimental studies consistently show the benefits of conjugated linoleic acid, in particular the *trans*-10, *cis*-12 isomer, which has metabolic benefits that include increased energy expenditure, decreased fat cell differentiation and proliferation, decreased fat synthesis, and increased fat burning and fat oxidation.[76]

• **Capsaicin**. The active agent in red pepper, capsaicin has been shown to enhance thermogenesis and energy metabolism in humans. In one study, energy expenditure was seen to increase in lean young women after consuming a capsaicin-rich curry.[77] Another study showed that consumption of a cultivar of red pepper increased core body temperature and metabolic rate in test humans.[78]

• **Extracts of ginger rich in gingerols**. These have been shown to increase oxygen consumption and enhance fat burning in experimental models.[79]

Pillar Number 7:
Restore Healthy Adipocyte (fat cell) Signaling

The adipocyte (fat cell) is the primary site for fat storage. Adipocytes of obese individuals are bloated with *triglycerides,* the form in which most fat exists in the body. Fat storage and release is tightly regulated by adipocyte *command signals.*

Weight gain occurs when adipocytes (fat cells) enlarge with large amounts of *triglycerides* due to overeating, nutrient deficiencies, excessive stress, and other causes. These factors, however, fail to address the reason why aging individuals put on fat pounds despite eating less, taking dietary supplements, and following other practices that should in theory lead to weight loss.

The aging process adversely affects the adipocyte *command signal* network, which helps explain the difficulty maturing individuals have in controlling their weight.

Adipocytes regulate their size and number by secreting *command signals.* Three important command *signals* that regulate adipocytes are:

- **Leptin**
- **Adiponectin**
- **Glycerol-3-phosphate dehydrogenase**

A seed extract of a common West African plant food called *Irvingia gabonensis* has been shown to favorably affect the three adipocyte command centers in the following ways:

LEPTIN

Released by adipocytes, **leptin** travels to the brain to perform two critical functions. First it signals the brain that enough food has been ingested and shuts down the appetite. It then depletes bloated adipocytes by promoting the burning of stored *triglycerides.* Leptin is much more abundant in the blood of obese individuals. The reason is that leptin receptor sites on cell membranes are inactivated by inflammatory factors in the body. **Irvingia** helps unblock "leptin resistance".

ADIPONECTIN

The second *command signal* released by *adipocytes* is adiponectin. The gene *transcription factors* associated with adiponectin help determine the amount of triglycerides stored in adipocytes and number of adipocytes formed in the body. Higher levels of adiponectin enhance insulin sensitivity, a long-established method to induce weight loss. Gene *transcriptional factors* involved with adiponectin are directly involved in sequential expression of adipocyte-specific proteins. ***Irvingia*** <u>suppresses</u> ***transcriptional factors*** involved in the formation of new adipocytes, while enhancing cell membrane insulin sensitivity by <u>increasing</u> ***adiponectin***. High circulating levels of **adiponectin** have been shown to protect against coronary artery disease whereas <u>low</u> adiponectin levels are observed in overweight individuals.

GLYCEROL-3-PHOSPHATE DEHYDROGENASE

An enzyme that facilitates the conversion of blood *glucose* into stored *triglyceride* fat is ***glycerol-3-phosphate dehydrogenase.*** The presence of this enzyme in the body reveals why low-fat diets alone fail to achieve sustained weight loss. The body will take ingested *carbohydrates* and convert them to stored triglyceride fat via the ***glycerol-3-phosphate dehydrogenase*** enzyme. **Irvingia** <u>inhibits</u> *glycerol-3-phosphate dehydrogenase,* thus reducing the amount of ingested sugars converted to body fat.

A clinical study has demonstrated significant weight loss of more than 20 lbs. over a 10-week period in response to taking a **150** mg ***Irvingia gabonensis*** extract twice daily. Study volunteers appeared to consume less calories in response to supplementation with the *Irvingia gabonensis* extract.[85]

You will read more about Irvingia in Chapter 3.

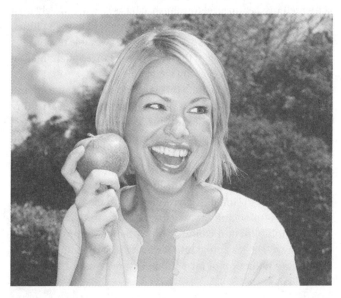

Pillar Number 8:
Inhibiting the Lipase Enzyme

Orlistat is an inhibitor of pancreatic and gastric lipase. It decreases the intestinal absorption of ingested dietary triglycerides by **30%**. By reducing the breakdown and absorption of dietary fat, orlistat enhances weight loss and lessens insulin resistance.

In studies of obese subjects, orlistat treatment improves *insulin* and *glucose* blood levels while significantly decreasing *C-reactive protein*, a marker for chronic inflammation. Orlistat treatment favorably influences other blood markers (such as *leptin* and *adiponectin*) involved with obesity.

In a one-year trial of overweight women, a group with metabolic syndrome treated with orlistat (120 mg, three times a day) and lifestyle modification lost 20.5 pounds compared with only 0.44 pounds weight loss in the placebo control group. A group of overweight women without metabolic syndrome taking the same dose of orlistat plus lifestyle modification lost **20.2** pounds more than the control group with metabolic syndrome.

In a three-month open-label trial of overweight patients without type 2 diabetes treated with orlistat (120 mg three times a day), men lost **17.4** pounds and women lost **12.3** pounds. In overweight patients with type 2 diabetes mellitus, men lost **18.7** pounds and women lost **12.5** pounds. In this study, leptin levels decreased by 51% in men with type 2 diabetes and 25% in women with type 2 diabetes mellitus. Leptin levels diminished by **48%** in overweight men and **23%** in overweight women without type 2 diabetes mellitus. Reduced leptin blood levels are considered a favorable response as they indicate a reduction in the "leptin resistance" phenomenon that often precludes successful weight loss.

Not all studies demonstrate this much weight loss in response to orlistat. Poor compliance is always a factor in the variability that exists among studies of the same compound. Another reason for these discrepancies is that orlistat users are warned to avoid excess ingestion of dietary fats and are likely to switch to consuming more simple carbohydrates. Overweight individuals often suffer metabolic disturbances, meaning that ingested sugars more readily convert to stored (triglyceride) fats on the body. So taking carbohydrate-blocking agents (special fibers and amylase/glucosidase inhibitors) in conjunction with orlistat for the first 90 days of a weight-loss program may be necessary to induce some immediate reduction of fat pounds that overweight and obese individuals expect.

Orlistat is available by prescription in **120** mg capsules as Xenical® or over-the-counter under the trade name **alli**® in **60** mg capsules. The suggested dose for the 90-day initiation period is **120** mg before each meal (three times a day). Make sure to take fat-soluble nutrients such as omega-3 fish oil, vitamins D, E, and K, and carotenoids (like lutein and zeaxanthin) at the time of the day furthest from the last orlistat dose, as its fat-blocking effects can interfere with absorption of these critical nutrients into the blood.[92,93]

Pillar Number 9:
Eat to Live a Long and Healthy Life

Don't embark on a weight-loss program by trying to follow a fad **diet** that can't be adhered to over the long term. Make *choices* as to what is more important, i.e., ingesting foods known to promote weight gain (and cause horrendous diseases) or selecting healthier foods that facilitate weight loss and protect against illness.

A little-known scientific fact about weight gain deals with ingestion of foods cooked at high temperatures (over 250 degrees). Overcooked foods damage our body's proteins while foods cooked at lower temperatures have been shown to facilitate weight loss.[100] So just changing how your foods are prepared could help you shed body fat and protect against age-related disease.

Conclusion

Solid scientific evidence shows that *excess* calorie ingestion accelerates the onset of degenerative disease <u>and</u> the aging process itself — in addition to promoting accumulation of **body fat.** It's never too late to change your lifestyle to promote better health and melt away excess body fat. Clinicians and patients truly committed to attaining a long and happy life will always include responsible diet and moderate exercise programs in their long-term plans.

If you have any questions on the scientific content of this book, please call a Life Extension Health Advisor at 1-866-820-8083.

References:
1. *Pharmacother.* 2001 Mar;35(3):314-28.
2. *Best Pract Res Clin Endocrinol Metab.* 2002 Dec;16(4):717-42.
3. *Curr Diabetes Rev.* 2008 Nov;4(4):340-56.
4. *J Am Diet Assoc.* 1998 Oct;98(10 Suppl 2):S23-6.
5. *Curr Diabetes Rev.* 2008 Nov;4(4):340-56.
6. *Am J Physiol Endocrinol Metab.* 2001 Sep;281(3):E626-32.
7. *Lipids Health Dis.* 2009 Mar 2;8:7.
8. *Altern Med Rev.* 2004 Mar;9(1):63-9.
9. *Integr Nutr.* 2008;11(2):15-21.
10. *Int J Med Sci.* 2007 Jan 24;4(1):45-52.
11. *Eur J Clin Invest.* 1994 Aug;24(Suppl 3):3-10.
12. http://www.innovactiv.com/en/pdf/Press_Release_InSea2_in_LEF_Enhanced_Irvingia-July_%202009.pdf
13. "A Pilot Study of the Effects of L-A/Cr: A Novel Combination of L-Arabinose and a Patented Chromium Supplement on Serum Glucose Levels After Sucrose Challenges," Gilbert R. Kaats, Ph.D., FACN; Harry Preuss, MD, MACN; Joel E. Michalek, Ph.D; Samuel C. Keith, BBA; Patti Keith, BBA; 2009.
14. *Nutrafoods.* 2008;7(4):21-8.
15. *J Nutr Biochem.* 2006 Jul;17(7):492-8.
16. *J Consult Clin Psychol.* 2003 Dec;71(6):1084-9.
17. *Intern Med.* 2007;46(9):543-6.
18. *J Amer College Nutr.* 45th Annual Meeting, Abs 77. (Long Beach, California.) 2004 Oct;76(2):272-5.
19. *Diabetes.* 1997 Nov;46(11):1786-91.
20. *Diabetes Care.* 2003 Apr;26(4):1147-52.
21. *Int J Circumpolar Health.* 2005 Sep;64(4):396-408.
22. *Am J Vet Res.* 2004 Aug;65(8):1090-9.
23. *Exp Clin Endocrinol Diabetes.* 2005 Feb;113(2):80-4.
24. *N Engl J Med.* 1996 Jan 25;334(4):269-70.
25. *Drugs.* 1999;58 Suppl 1:71-3.
26. *Eur J Clin Invest.* 1998 Jun;28(6):441-6.
27. *Diabetes.* 1986 Feb;35(2):155-64.
28. *Diabetes Care.* 2006 Jun;29(6):1337-44.
29. *J Gerontol A Biol Sci Med Sci.* 1995 May;50(3):B142-7.
30. *Obes Surg.* 2005 Apr;15(4):462-73.
31. *Am J Clin Nutr.* 1992 Jul;56(1 Suppl):179S-81S.
32. *J Clin Endocrinol Metab.* 2002 Oct;87(10):4522-7.
33. *Aging Male.* 2002 Jun;5(2):98-102.
34. *Eur J Med.* 1992 Oct;1(6):329-36.
35. *JAMA.* 2004 Nov 10;292(18):2243-8.
36. *Obes Rev.* 2004 Nov;5(4):197-216.
37. *Int J Obes Relat Metab Disord.* 1996 Apr;20(4):291-302.
38. *Med Hypotheses.* 2002 Jun;58(6):487-90.
39. http://www.ars.usda.gov/research/publications/publications.htm?SEQ_NO_115=181996. Accessed October 9, 2009.
40. *Am J Clin Nutr.* 2003 Nov;78(5):920-7.
41. *Int J Obesity Relat Metab Disord.* 1998 May;22(5):454-60.
42. *JAMA.* 1999 Oct 27;282(16):1539-46.
43. *Int J ObeS Relat Metab Disord.* 2001 Mar;25(3):301-6.
44. *Am J Ther.* 2007 Mar;14(2):203-12.
45. *Asia Pac J Clin Nutr.* 2007;16(1):16-24.
46. http://www.cspinet.org/new/sugar_limit.html
47. *Journal of Nutrition* 2001; 131: 79b-799.
48. A Pilot Study of the Effects of L-A/Cr: A Novel Combination of L-Arabinose and a Patented Chromium Supplement on Serum Glucose Levels After Sucrose Challenges," Gilbert R. Kaats, Ph.D., FACN; Harry Preuss, MD, MACN; Joel E. Michalek, Ph.D; Samuel C. Keith, BBA; Patti Keith, BBA; 2009.
49. *Am J Med.* 2007 Sep;120(9 Suppl 1):S10-6.
50. *Nature.* 2006 Dec 14;444(7121):881-7.
51. *Am J Med.* 2007 Feb;120(2 Suppl 1):S3-S8.
52. *Curr Alzheimer Res.* 2007 Apr;4(2):117-22.

53. *Am J Clin Nutr.* 2007 Jul;86(1):48-54.
54. *Metabolism.* 2007 May;56(5):614-22.
55. *Int J Obes Relat Metab Disord.* 2003 Mar;27(3):347-54.
56. *Coron Artery Dis.* 2007 Sep;18(6):433-6.
57. *Gastroenterology.* 2003 Jan;124(1):71-9.
58. *Diabetes.* 2002 Jun;51(6):1889-95.
59. *Acta Physiol* (Oxf). 2008 Jan;192(1):127-35.
60. Lemberg R. Ed., Oryx Press; 1998:51.
61. *Am J Clin Nutr.* 2003 May;77(5):1112-8.
62. *Curr Drug Metab.* 2007 Apr;8(3):289-95.
63. *J Clin Invest.* 2003 Dec;112(12):1821-30.
64. *Eat Weight Disord.* 1997 Dec;2(4):211-5.
65. *Int J Eating Disord.* 1985:4(3):281-92.
66. *Exp Gerontol.* 2007 Nov 21.
67. *Circulation.* 2002 Feb 19;105(7):804-9.
68. *Curr Vasc Pharmacol.* 2007 Oct;5(4):249-58.
69. *Int J Obes Relat Metab Disord.* 2004 Aug;28(8):998-1003.
70. *Pflugers Arch.* 2007 Sep 29.
71. *J Am Coll Cardiol.* 2004 Mar 17;43(6):1056-61.
72. *Am J Cardiol.* 2007 Feb 19;99(4A):68B-79B.
73. *Am J Clin Nutr.* 1999 Dec;70(6):1040-5.
74. *Int J Obes Relat Metab Disord.* 2000 Feb;24(2):252-8.
75. *Mol Nutr Food Res.* 2008 Jun;52(6):631-45.
76. *Int J Obes Relat Metab Disord.* 2004 Aug;28(8):941-55.
77. *J Nutr Sci Vitaminol* (Tokyo). 2000 Dec;46(6):309-15.
78. *Biosci Biotechnol Biochem.* 2001 Sep;65(9):2033-6.
79. *Int J Obes Relat Metab Disord.* 1992 Oct;16(10):755-63.
80. *BMJ.* 2007 Dec 1;335(7630):1134.
81. *Am J Epidemiol.* 2007 Oct 15;166(8):932-40.
82. *Eur J Gastroenterol Hepatol.* 2007 Aug;19(8):623-30.
83. *J Nutr.* 2007 Jan;137(1 Suppl):161S-9.
84. *Cancer.* 1991 May 15;67(10):2622-5.
85. *Lipids Health Dis.* 2009 Mar 2;8:7.
86. *J Am Soc Nephrol.* 2006 Apr;17(4 Suppl 2):S109-11.
87. *Arq Bras Endocrinol Metabol.* 2005 Apr;49(2):196-204.
88. *Asia Pac J Clin Nutr.* 2007;16(4):671-6.
89. *Am J Clin Nutr.* 2007 Nov;86(5):1293-301.
90. *Obesity* (Silver Spring). 2007 Jun;15(6):1473-83.
91. *J Appl Physiol.* 2005 Oct;99(4):1613-8.
92. *Ann Pharmacother.* 2001 Mar;35(3):314-28.
93. *Pharmacotherapy.* 2000 Mar;20(3):270-9.
94. *Curr Gastroenterol Rep.* 2005 Dec;7(6):451-4.
95. *Int J Eat Disord.* 2006 Sep;39(6):492-7.
96. *J Immigr Minor Health.* 2007 Dec 9 [Epub ahead of print].
97. *Angiology.* 2007 Feb-Mar;58(1):102-5.
98. *Wien Klin Wochenschr.* 2006 Sep;118(17-18):558-61.
99. *J Am Diet Assoc.* 2007 Mar;107(3):441-7.
100. *Free Radic Bio Med.* 28, 1708-1716 (2000).

CHAPTER 2

How Proper Blood Testing Can Help You Safely Shed Fat Pounds

The prevalence of obesity has doubled since **1980.** The latest study reveals that for the first time **obese** Americans outnumber those who are merely **overweight.**

The war against obesity is an obvious failure. Overlooked are a plethora of research findings indicating **substantial fat-loss** effects in response to the proper use of **bioidentical hormones,** certain **prescription drugs** and **nutrients**, along with **lifestyle changes.**

The reason these **proven weight-loss strategies** have not caught on is that when used in isolation, they often fail to meet the **expectations** of a typical obese or overweight individual.

This eye-opening chapter discusses how your doctor can interpret **blood test results** to prescribe an armada of medications, natural hormones, and lifestyle alterations that can safely induce substantial and sustainable weight loss.

Our Bloated Bloodstreams

Overeating is associated with *bloating* of the gastrointestinal tract (stomach and intestines). What happens *after* excess fats and sugars leave the digestive system and enter the bloodstream seems to have been forgotten.

People in modern societies have succumbed to a pathological propensity of ingesting *excess* calories throughout the day (and sometimes night). The result is that our bloodstreams are chronically *bloated* with fats and sugars. Constant exposure to excess fats and sugars results in insulin resistance,[1-3] oxidative stress,[4,5] vascular inflammation,[1,5-9] and platelet activation[10] ... all of which sharply increase heart attack,[1,2,6,11] stroke,[6] and diabetes[12,13] risks. Chronically *bloated* bloodstreams also contribute to unwanted weight gain and preclude shedding surplus fat pounds.

A growing number of medical studies discuss the role of *postprandial lipemia* (too much **fat** remaining in the blood after a meal) and *postprandial hyperglycemia* (too much after-meal **glucose**) as culprits in today's obesity epidemic. As long as our meals contain enough of the wrong fats, a transient increase in **postprandial lipemia** will likely occur. Even when simple carbohydrates are avoided, *insulin resistance* causes many aging people to suffer higher-than-desirable blood **glucose** and correspondingly elevated **triglyceride** levels.[14,15]

Unless definitive actions are taken, most people will spend most of the day in a *postprandial* state, i.e., their bloodstreams chronically overloaded with sugars and fats. One might think that dieting alone would resolve postprandial metabolic disorders. But there are fundamental age-related impediments that often require *pharmaceutical* intervention.

Dietary Sugars or Fats — There May be Little Difference

Postprandial metabolic disorders can be caused by chronically eating the wrong kinds of fats or simple carbohydrates. It may not matter which food groups are restricted. The blood becomes so saturated with fats or sugars that enzymatic conversions of fat to glucose and vice versa results in *chronic postprandial overload* that can sabotage the best-laid weight-loss plan.

Most of us are familiar with how delayed or excess insulin secretion *(postprandial hyperinsulinemia)* contributes to weight gain. Consuming soluble fiber <u>before</u> each meal can help normalize insulin responses and the release of dietary carbohydrates into the bloodstream. Correcting the postprandial disorders afflicting overweight and obese individuals, however, often requires *more* aggressive intervention.

Please know that even with so-called *normal* <u>fasting</u> glucose and triglyceride blood levels, your glucose and triglyceride levels can remain elevated in your bloodstream for two-to-eight hours after eating.

Temporarily Suppressing Fat and Carbohydrate Enzymes

In recognizing *postprandial disorders* as an underlying cause of weight gain and impediment to successful fat loss, we will review studies showing benefits when *lipase, alpha-glucosidase,* or *alpha-amylase* enzymes are inhibited in the digestive tract.

For some people, drugs or nutrients that inhibit these digestive enzymes will cause gastrointestinal discomforts. The objective of using these *enzyme inhibitors* on a 90-day trial basis is to provide you with an opportunity to restore a healthier metabolic profile, provide immediate fat-loss effects (especially in the abdomen), and educate you about life-long dietary patterns that should be followed.

The temporary use of compounds that inhibit fat and sugar absorption is designed to "break" the "food addiction" cycle. For example, if your diet consists of more than 30% calories from fat, a *lipase* inhibitor drug (orlistat) will induce unpleasant gastrointestinal side effects and provide strong motivation to make healthier food choices.[16]

Treating Postprandial Disorders

It is difficult to initiate weight loss in the presence of a bloodstream chronically overloaded with glucose and triglycerides. While each person will express individual variability, implementing a treatment regimen to reduce the postprandial burden will help improve metabolic parameters that help reduce body fat, while lowering markers of vascular disease risk.

Everyone, of course, is encouraged to initiate diets low in saturated and omega-6 fats, while consuming complex whole-food carbohydrates and soluble and insoluble fiber, along with foods that naturally contain omega-3 fatty acids. Most people, however, require additional interventions to ameliorate postprandial disorders developed over years or decades.

The <u>four</u> steps for *reversing* postprandial overload are:

1. Reduce calorie intake, especially saturated fats, omega-6 fats, and simple sugars.
2. Block acute glucose absorption to reduce excess insulin response.
3. Inhibit *lipase, alpha-amylase,* and *alpha-glucosidase* enzymes to reduce amount of absorbed fat and carbohydrate calories.
4. Modulate hormones and enzyme systems in the liver, blood, and adipose tissues to induce healthy metabolism and removal of excess fats-glucose from the bloodstream and stored triglycerides from abdominal adipocytes.

Inhibiting the *Alpha-Glucosidase* Enzyme

Postprandial hyperglycemia is a characteristic feature of insulin resistance. Excess blood *glucose* rapidly converts into *triglycerides* and other lipids and impairs fat clearance with the result being *postprandial lipemia.*[17] Excessive *postprandial* absorption of glucose has been associated with greater cardiovascular disease risk than the *fasting* plasma glucose level.[18,19]

Aggressive actions to suppress *postprandial hyperglycemia* are an important first step in reducing excess body fat <u>and</u> protecting against vascular disease.

Before carbohydrates are absorbed from food, they must be broken down into smaller sugar particles like glucose by enzymes in the small intestine. One of the enzymes involved is *alpha-glucosidase*. By inhibiting this enzyme, simple carbohydrates (like sucrose) are not broken down as efficiently and glucose absorption is delayed. *Alpha-glucosidase inhibitors* are available as prescription drugs (such as *acarbose*) or dietary supplements (such as InSea²™). They function by <u>decreasing</u> the breakdown of simple carbohydrates in the intestine, resulting in a slower and lower rise in blood glucose throughout the day, especially after meals.

A multicenter, placebo-controlled randomized trial revealed that the *alpha-glucosidase* inhibitor drug acarbose improved *postprandial hyperglycemia* and reduced the risk of development of type 2 diabetes in patients with impaired glucose tolerance. In this study, acarbose treatment was also found to slow the progression of *intima-media thickness* of the carotid arteries, a surrogate marker for atherosclerosis, and reduce the incidence of cardiovascular diseases and newly diagnosed hypertension. This study also showed that acarbose produced small reductions in body mass index and waist circumference.[20]

A meta-analysis of seven long-term studies has also shown that intervention with acarbose prevents heart attack and cardiovascular diseases in type 2 diabetic patients. This analysis showed improvements in glucose control, triglyceride levels, body weight, and systolic blood pressure in response to acarbose treatment.[21]

How Effective Are *Alpha-Glucosidase* Inhibitors?

An overview of the published literature on *alpha-glucosidase* inhibitors reveals the following:

INDICATOR	EFFICACY
Reducing Postprandial Hyperglycemia	Very Effective
Improving Cardiac Risk Factors	Very Effective
Preventing Heart Attack	Very Effective
Inducing Body Fat Loss	Minimally Effective

It is regrettable that the medical establishment has largely ignored the multiple benefits demonstrated by *alpha-glucosidase* inhibitors in published clinical trials. One study showed a 91% reduction in acute heart attack incidence in response to acarbose therapy in patients with impaired glucose tolerance.[22] A meta-analysis showed a 36% decreased incidence of type 2 diabetes in patients taking acarbose.[23]

You would think these kinds of studies would make headline news, but pharmaceutical companies have not promoted these findings the way they do for statin drugs. One reason may be that the public can access low-cost *alpha-glucosidase inhibitors* as over-the-counter dietary supplements or low-cost generic drugs.

The weight loss shown in response to *alpha-glucosidase* inhibitors is considerably less than what one might expect. While one report showed a **15.4-pound** weight loss over five months in a single case study, most clinical studies show weight loss of only a few pounds.[23] Based on these reports, *alpha-glucosidase* inhibitors (like acarbose) should not be used as standalone methods for inducing weight loss. *Alpha-glucosidase* inhibitors have been documented to effectively ameliorate postprandial conditions[24,25] and would appear to be an important initial constituent in a comprehensive weight-loss program. But a multi-pronged approach is *required* to successfully combat obesity.

Additional Benefits Using *Alpha-Amylase* Inhibitors

Carbohydrates contribute to the synthesis of fats in our bodies. Since *postprandial hyperglycemia* leads to an increase in fat storage, the use of substances that interfere with glucose break-down and absorption are important components of a weight-loss program.

As previously noted in Chapter 1 (Pillar 3), an extract from the white kidney bean (*Phaseolus vulgaris*) targets the *alpha-amylase* enzyme and helps reduce the rapid increase in blood glucose after consumption of a carbohydrate-rich meal. And *L-arabinose* targets the sucrase enzyme, helping to delay the rapid rise in blood sugar associated with sucrose consumption.

Anyone with a fasting triglyceride blood level over **80** mg/dL should be suspected to be suffering some degree of *postprandial lipemia*. Overweight patients usually present with fasting triglyceride readings well over **150** mg/dL, which indicates postprandial *hyperglycemia* and *lipemia* as underlying causes of their weight gain. Inhibiting carbohydrate absorption will help reduce triglyceride and glucose blood levels.

As stated in the previous chapter, medications and nutrients shown to be effective in blunting the sharp glucose/insulin surge in response to ingestion of dietary carbohydrates include:

Beta-glucan (soluble fiber powder) .... 5–10 grams
Acarbose (generic prescription drug) .... 50–100 mg
Metformin (generic prescription drug) ... 250–850 mg
Phase 3™ (*L-arabinose*) .... 550 mg
Phase 2™ (white kidney bean extact) .... 445 mg

Inhibiting the Lipase Enzyme

A regrettable consequence of normal aging is that people no longer have the *metabolic capacity* to consume the same number of calories they did in their youth. Part of this loss of metabolic capacity relates to the aging patient's increasing *inability* to rapidly utilize and then purge dietary fats from their bloodstream.

Excess calorie intakes manifest outwardly as unwanted fat deposits. The *vascular* and *inflammatory* damage inflicted by chronic overeating, however, can be as deadly as when a smoker diagnosed with *emphysema* continues to smoke.

We fear "food addiction" may be an even greater problem based on startling studies that began appearing only a few years ago. These studies show heart attack and stroke risks to be substantially higher in patients with only *modestly* elevated after-meal (postprandial) *triglyceride* levels.[30] Coupled with data revealing how obesity is related to chronically elevated blood fat levels (lipemia), it is critical to take aggressive steps to reduce the amount of <u>fats</u> that linger in patients' bloodstreams.

The section following this describes a number of proven methods to reduce *postprandial lipemia*. Overweight and obese patients seeking to lose substantial body fat, however, may consider a 90-day regimen using the *lipase inhibitor* drug **orlistat.**

Orlistat reduces dietary fat absorption by **30%** and has been around for about 11 years.[31,32] It functions by blocking an enzyme (lipase) that breaks down dietary fat in the intestinal tract, thus impeding its absorption into the bloodstream.

Clinical studies demonstrate significant weight loss in response to using this drug.[33,34] In the real world, however, orlistat has been associated with fat-laden diarrhea and fat seepage into patients' underwear, causing patients to discontinue its use.

We are concerned with the unpleasant potential side effects of orlistat, but we are even more frightened about the inability of obese individuals to lose enough weight to regain youthful metabolic function. We therefore suggest that you consider taking orlistat for 60–90 days. It will dramatically <u>reduce</u> *postprandial lipemia*.

How Orlistat Works

Orlistat is an inhibitor of pancreatic and gastric lipase. It decreases the intestinal absorption of ingested dietary triglycerides by 30%.[35]

By reducing *postprandial lipemia,* orlistat enhances weight loss, lessens insulin resistance, and improves cardiovascular risk factors in patients with metabolic syndrome, with and without type 2 diabetes.[36]

In studies of obese subjects, orlistat treatment improves *insulin* and *glucose* blood levels while significantly decreasing *C-reactive protein,* a marker of chronic inflammation.[37-39] Orlistat treatment favorably influences other blood markers (such as *leptin* and *adiponectin*) that are involved with obesity.[38]

Short-term (10 days) use of orlistat reduced daytime *lipemia* (triglyceridemia) by 17% in obese, non-diabetic women with metabolic syndrome, with only minimal side effects.[40]

In a one-year trial of overweight women, a group with metabolic syndrome treated with orlistat (120 mg three times a day) and lifestyle modification lost **20.5** lbs compared with only **0.44** lbs weight loss in the placebo control group.[43] A group of overweight women without metabolic syndrome taking the same dose of orlistat plus lifestyle modification lost 20.2 lbs more than the control group with metabolic syndrome.[43]

In a three-month open-label trial of overweight patients without type 2 diabetes treated with orlistat (120 mg three times a day), men lost 17.4 lbs and women lost 12.3 lbs.[40] In overweight patients with type 2 diabetes mellitus, men lost 18.7 lbs and women lost 12.5 lbs.[44] In overweight patients without type 2 diabetes mellitus, the level of insulin resistance as measured by HOMA-IR (a validated modeling instrument for insulin resistance) decreased by **28%** with orlistat treatment.[44] For overweight patients with type 2 diabetes mellitus, insulin resistance decreased by **41%.** Leptin levels decreased by **51%** in men with type 2 diabetes and **29%** in women with type 2 diabetes mellitus. Leptin levels dropped by **49%** in overweight men and **28%** in overweight women without type 2 diabetes mellitus.[44] A reduction in leptin blood levels is considered a favorable response as it indicates a reduction in the "leptin resistance" phenomenon that so often precludes weight loss.

Not all studies demonstrate this much weight loss in response to orlistat.[41,42] Poor compliance is always a factor in the variability. Another reason for these discrepancies is that orlistat users are warned to avoid excess ingestion of dietary fats, and are likely to switch to consuming more simple carbohydrates. Overweight individuals often suffer metabolic disturbances, meaning ingested sugars readily convert to stored (triglyceride) fats on the body. So taking carbohydrate-blocking agents (*alpha-glucosidase* and *alpha-amylase inhibitors*) in <u>conjunction</u> with **orlistat** for the first 60–90 days may be necessary to induce immediate reduction of fat pounds.

In conjunction with the medications, dietary alterations, supplements, and lifestyle changes discussed in this article, the use of orlistat for a 60- to 90-day initiation period should provide some immediate weight loss, while enabling the re-establishment of a more youthful metabolic profile in the body whereby *postprandial lipemia*, insulin resistance, and other metabolic abnormalities are suppressed.

Orlistat is available by prescription in **120** mg capsules as **Xenical®**, or over-the-counter under the trade name **alli®** in **60** mg capsules. The suggested dose for the initial 60–90 day initiation period is **120** mg before each meal (three times a day). Considering the relatively high cost of over-the-counter **alli®**, patients with insurance coverage might save money by using prescription-strength orlistat.

Restoring Youthful Metabolic Parameters From the Inside

At this point, you have erected a multi-pronged <u>barrier</u> to impede the excess <u>absorption</u> of unwanted calories. These include:

1. Reducing the intake of simple carbohydrates, saturated fats, omega-6 fats, and trans fats.
2. Impeding rapid surges in glucose and insulin release from excess carbohydrate ingestion by inhibiting the *alpha-glucosidase* and *alpha-amylase* enzymes (using the drug acarbose and the nutrients Phase 2™, and Phase 3™).
3. Suppressing the *insulin spike* by slowing carbohydrate absorption with soluble fiber taken before each meal.
4. Inhibiting fat absorption by taking the *lipase inhibitor* orlistat.

For many people, sticking to the above program for the period we suggest should provide optimal fat-loss benefits. We prefer that most people not use orlistat for more than 90 days. But people successfully benefiting from orlistat may continue it longer.

The 90-day program we have suggested will dramatically *reverse* many of the metabolic imbalances that are underlying causes of excess fat accumulation and increased vascular disease risk. Overweight and obese individuals can expect to see a rapid reduction in

(Continued on page 33)

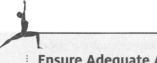

Ensure Adequate Absorption of Fat-Soluble Nutrients in Orlistat Patients

A concern with taking a lipase-inhibiting drug like **orlistat** is reduced absorption of fat-soluble vitamins. Since orlistat only reduces fat absorption by 30%, a patient taking supplemental vitamin A, D, E, and K should be able to maintain more than sufficient levels of these nutrients.

The body has a significant capacity to store **vitamin A,** so we would not expect a problem with this nutrient.

Vitamin D is also stored rather well. However, an obese patient might consider taking **10,000 IU** each day of vitamin D for one week prior to initiating orlistat to build up sufficient levels. Obese individuals require more vitamin D than lean people. This nutrient also has functions that may help facilitate weight loss.[161-163] Vitamin D status can be assessed with a blood test that measures 25-hydroxy-vitamin D. Optimal blood levels are **50–80 ng/mL** of **25-hydroxy-vitamin D**. Patients should be able to maintain these levels by supplementing with **5,000** to **10,000** IU of **vitamin D3** at the time of the day that is most removed from their last **orlistat** dose.

Vitamin K, an important fat-soluble vitamin, is not stored well by the body. The ideal form of vitamin K2 is **menaquinone-7,** which remains in the body several days after ingestion. The minimum suggested daily dose of **menaquinone-7** vitamin K2 is **90 mcg,** and can be taken in supplements that also provide **vitamin K1** and the **menaquinone-4** form of vitamin K2. Like vitamin D3, vitamin K should be taken at the time of the day furthest from the patient's last orlistat dose. (Those taking the anticoagulant drug Coumadin® [warfarin] must use extreme caution if supplementing with vitamin K and may consider using a low dose of this vitamin [45 mcg of menaquinone-7 a day] <u>only</u> under the close supervision of the physician prescribing warfarin.)

Ingesting optimal amounts of **omega-3 fats** is critical in reducing *postprandial lipemia.*[164-165] Patients should consume at least **1,400** mg of **eicosapentaenoic acid (EPA)** and **1,000** mg of **docosahexaenoic acid (DHA)** in a fish oil supplement. Those with triglyceride levels above 99 mg/dL of blood often require more EPA/DHA. Omega-3 **fish oil** supplements should be taken with vitamins D and K.

Fat-soluble carotenoids such as **zeaxanthin, lutein,** and **beta-carotene,** along with alpha and **gamma tocopherol** should also be taken (usually at bedtime) furthest from the patient's last orlistat dose. Fat-soluble nutrients in a multivitamin can be taken with orlistat but at a time most removed from their last orlistat dose.

body weight and abdominal inches that will incent you to follow a reduced-calorie regimen with Mediterranean diet-type food choices and plenty of dietary fiber.

The long-term objective is to *restore* a more youthful metabolic pattern that will last a lifetime. This most often requires hormonal balancing and enzymatic modulation at the cellular level. For men, replacing free *testosterone* lost to normal aging is usually required. Women deficient in *estrogen* are encouraged to restore estrogen to more desirable ranges. Both sexes should maintain TSH (thyroid-stimulating hormone) and T3 (tri-iodothyronine) *thyroid* hormone levels in the optimal ranges described later in this article.

Normal aging results in reduced insulin signaling throughout the body that disrupts healthy glucose metabolism. The prescription drug *metformin* helps correct several mechanisms involved in glucose impairment by increasing insulin sensitivity, enhancing peripheral glucose uptake in energy-producing cells, decreasing intestinal absorption of glucose, and suppressing excess glucose synthesis from the liver.[45-47] Metformin also increases a satiety hormone called *glucagon-like peptide 1,* thus helping induce a long-term appetite-suppressing effect that will better enable adjustment to a life-long reduced-calorie diet.[48,49]

Effects of Sex Hormones on Adipose Tissues

Sex hormones are involved in the metabolism, accumulation, and distribution of body fat. Adipocytes (fat cells) have receptors to bind testosterone, estrogen, and progesterone, thus enabling these sex hormones to exert a direct action.

Sex steroid hormones carry out their function in adipose tissues by both genomic and non-genomic mechanisms.[74] In the genomic mechanism, the sex steroid hormone binds to its receptor on the adipocyte and can regulate the transcription of genes involved in obesity. *Leptin* is a hormone secreted from adipocytes that regulates appetite and induces beneficial triglyceride breakdown in adipocytes. *Lipoprotein lipase* is an enzyme that breaks down circulating triglycerides into free fatty acids that are readily stored in adipocytes (fat cells). Both *leptin* and *lipoprotein lipase* exert control over adipose (fat) tissues and are *genomically* regulated by *sex hormones*.

In the non-genomic mechanism, sex hormones can activate certain *hormone-sensitive lipases,* ultimately leading to lipolysis (fat breakdown). In the presence of certain sex hormones, a normal distribution of body fat exists. On the other hand, with an imbalance of certain sex hormones (as occurs with aging), there is a tendency towards an increase in abdominal obesity: a major risk factor for cardiovascular disease,[75,76] type 2 diabetes,[77] and cancer.[76,78-80]

Since sex hormones regulate the amount and distribution of adipose tissues, they are key elements of a comprehensive program to eliminate obesity. When properly prescribed, bioidentical hormone replacement therapy in postmenopausal women and men often reduces the degree of abdominal obesity.[74,81-83]

Testosterone Prevents Triglycerides from Accumulating in the Male Abdomen

In men, a testosterone *deficit* is often accompanied by visceral obesity. When deficient men are supplemented with testosterone, the result is a region-specific decrease in the visceral (abdominal) adipose tissue mass.[74,84] This suggests that testosterone is exerting its effects by inhibiting lipid uptake and/or enhancing lipid mobilization from adipocytes, particularly abdominal fatty tissues.

To assess the effect of testosterone on fat mass, a study was done using labeled triglyceride fatty acids and measuring their incorporation into adipose tissues in two different regions of the body. The study subjects were all abdominally obese and divided into three groups. Group one received topical natural *testosterone* cream, the second group received a testosterone metabolite called dihydrotestosterone, while the third group was given a placebo cream. After two months, the testosterone group exhibited a **34%** reduction in triglyceride *uptake* and increased *turnover* rate of triglycerides in abdominal adipose tissue.[85]

Interestingly, the uptake of labeled *triglyceride* at baseline was **20%** greater in *abdominal* fat compared with *upper leg* fat, which helps explain why so many men suffer expanding waistlines as they age, especially in the presence of low testosterone. This study shows that testosterone replacement *diminished* triglyceride uptake by fat cells in the abdomen, while simultaneously *promoting* a more rapid release of abdominal triglyceride stores.[85]

The underlying mechanism proposed by the study's authors was a significant **47%** decrease in *lipoprotein lipase* activity in the abdominal region. As discussed earlier, lipoprotein lipase is involved in the deposition of triglycerides in adipocytes, thus causing fat cells (and people) to become bloated.

Triglyceride is the predominant form of fat that bloats adipocytes. Excess fat in the bloodstream after eating (postprandial lipemia) is often described as *postprandial hypertriglyceridemia*. Interestingly, testosterone supplementation can reduce blood triglyceride levels

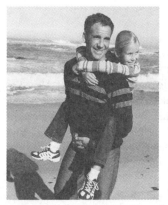

by increasing their breakdown in the liver (via increased *hepatic lipase activity*). Testosterone also improves insulin sensitivity and can facilitate a reduction in *postprandial hyperglycemia*.[86] Several additional mechanisms have been identified that enable testosterone to reduce triglyceride levels in abdominal adipocytes (fat cells) of men.[85,87]

A number of studies document a reduction in belly fat after men with low testosterone are supplemented with testosterone.[88-90] If a blood test reveals a less-than-optimal *free testosterone* level (<u>below</u> 20 pg/mL), consider asking your doctor to prescribe a **topical testosterone cream** after first ruling out prostate cancer using a PSA (prostate-specific antigen) blood test and digital rectal exam. *(Refer to the sidebar "How to Safely Restore Youthful Testosterone in Aging Men" on page 42 for prescribing information.)*

Some men will convert (aromatize) too much of their testosterone to estrogen. Optimal estradiol levels in men range from **20 to 30** pg/mL of blood at the time of this writing.[91-92] Excess estradiol can be easily suppressed by asking your doctor to prescribe an aromatase-inhibiting drug like **Arimidex®** in the dose of **0.5** mg two times a week.

Make sure that estradiol levels are not lowered below **20** pg/mL of blood as this may disable testosterone's ability to induce abdominal fat loss. Some studies suggest that the <u>decrease</u> in abdominal *lipoprotein lipase* that occurs in response to testosterone replacement therapy may have to do with the conversion of some of the testosterone to estrogen.[93] These studies are contradicted when observing abdominally obese men whose blood tests reveal low free testosterone and excess estradiol. These overweight men often present with enlarged breasts (gynecomastia) induced by this excess estradiol. Since much of the excess estradiol in these aging men is a result of the aromatization of testosterone to estradiol in abdominal adipocytes, it is difficult to comprehend that testosterone's benefit in reducing belly fat is reliant on significant aromatization to estradiol.

These subtle nuances, which vary considerably amongst individuals, are why regular **blood testing** to ensure optimal *free testosterone* and *estrogen* levels is so important.

(Continued on page 39)

Natural and Pharmaceutical Methods to Reduce Postprandial Lipemia

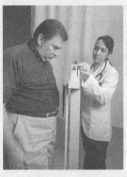 Overweight and obese individuals demonstrate chronically elevated **fat** levels in their blood long after meals are ingested. This **postprandial lipemia** is a significant risk factor for degenerative disease and can sabotage efforts to reverse type 2 diabetes, metabolic syndrome, and obesity.

Saturated fats, like those found in butter, shortening, and fried foods, are especially potent inducers of excess postprandial lipoproteins. Because postprandial disorders cause fats to linger longer, avoiding unhealthy fats is doubly important. Minimizing these fats also reduces LDL, blood pressure, inflammation, and cancer risk. While avoiding saturated fats will not eliminate postprandial lipids and lipoproteins, it will help reduce them.[50] A polyunsaturated omega-6 fatty acid derived from safflower also raises postprandial lipid and lipoprotein levels, just as saturated fats do.[51,52]

Although the immediate cause of persistent and increased postprandial lipoproteins is an unhealthy fat-containing meal, two varieties of fat <u>reduce</u> postprandial lipoproteins:

• Monounsaturated oils, like **olive oil,** modestly reduce postprandial lipoproteins. Monounsaturated oils may thus be a preferable form of oil for cooking and everyday use.[52,53]

• Polyunsaturated **omega-3** fatty acids reduce postprandial lipoproteins dramatically.[51] Sources of omega-3 fatty acids include fish oil, flaxseed oil, and walnuts.

• Although undesirable saturated fats lead to increased postprandial lipoprotein particles, a low-fat diet does not reduce postprandial lipoproteins. All too often, low-fat diets can evolve into diets rich in processed carbohydrates, which cause postprandial lipid and lipoprotein particles to multiply out of control.[54] Diets rich in monounsaturated fats, omega-3 fats, fiber, and lean proteins, and low in saturated fats and processed carbohydrates, are effective tools in reducing postprandial lipoproteins.[55]

The following strategies can <u>reduce</u> **triglycerides** dramatically and help reduce or eliminate elevated postprandial fats:

- **Weight loss** can greatly reduce triglycerides and postprandial lipids and lipoproteins, particularly when accomplished with a diet low in fiber-poor, refined carbohydrates and high in fiber, lean protein, and monounsaturated fats. Cutting out processed carbohydrates (breads, crackers, breakfast cereals, bagels, pretzels made with refined, processed white flour) alone can yield a **30%** <u>reduction</u> in postprandial lipoproteins.[56,57] Increasing intake of yogurt, cottage cheese, and other low-fat dairy products, raw almonds and walnuts, and fish, chicken, turkey, and other sources of lean protein will also help. Weight loss restores the insulin responsiveness lost in metabolic syndrome, which also reduces postprandial lipids and lipoproteins.[58]

- **Omega-3 fatty acids** in fish oil exert powerful effects in reducing postprandial lipoproteins. Ingesting just 1,200 mg of EPA/DHA from fish oil can easily lower postprandial fat remnants **50%,** and higher doses produce even greater reductions. When fasting triglycerides are higher than 80–99 mg/dL, higher doses of fish oil may be indicated. Omega-3 fatty acids decrease the liver's production of artery-damaging very low-density lipoprotein (VLDL) by 30% or more.[59,60] Fish oil can safely augment the cholesterol-lowering effects of statin drugs such as Lipitor®, yielding dramatic improvement in triglycerides, VLDL, and postprandial lipoproteins.[61]

- **Soy protein** (20 grams per day) from tofu, soy milk, soy protein powder, and other sources can lower LDL by 10–20 mg/dL and reduce postprandial lipoproteins by 10%.[62] We suggest soy as part of a healthy diet in which it is substituted for unhealthy fats in meat.

- **Green tea** contains catechins (flavonoids) that can decrease postprandial lipids and lipoproteins by up to **30%**.[63] Approximately 600–700 mg of green tea catechins are required to achieve this effect, the equivalent of 6–12 servings of brewed tea. Nutritional supplements provide green tea catechins at this dose. Green tea's effectiveness in accelerating weight loss may in part relate to its ability to reduce postprandial lipids and lipoproteins. For green tea to be effective, it should be taken immediately before meals to help block the absorption of fats and sugars. Use decaffeinated green tea extract supplements if caffeine bothers you.

(Continued next page)

A new **green tea phytosome** that will be described later in this book has demonstrated remarkable weight loss and triglyceride-lowering effects at a dose of only 300 mg a day.

- **Vigorous exercise** can reduce postprandial lipoproteins by 30%.[64]

- **Niacin** in doses of **2,000** to **3,000 mg** a day will significantly lower triglycerides, and provide beneficial changes in HDL while changing LDL particles to a less atherogenic form.[65,66] Niacin can cause a skin "flushing" side effect that can be mitigated by using a "no-flush" niacin supplement.

- **Diabetes treatment** (with insulin or oral hypoglycemic drugs) significantly reduces postprandial lipoprotein levels.[67,68] The thiazolidinedione drug Actos® may be especially effective.[69] The drug metformin also reduces fasting and postprandial triglycerides by 25%.[70] (Caution: Like other thiazolidinediones, Actos® can cause fluid retention, which may lead to or exacerbate heart failure. Actos® should be discontinued if any deterioration in cardiac status occurs.)

- **Statin drugs** such as generic simvastatin, Crestor®, and Lipitor® not only lower cholesterol, but also can reduce postprandial lipoproteins by 30–80%.[71]

- **Fibrates** (cholesterol-lowering drugs such as Lopid® and Lofibra®) can reduce postprandial lipids and lipoproteins by 70%. They can be a useful second-line strategy if fish oil, weight loss, and nutritional efforts fail to do the job.[72]

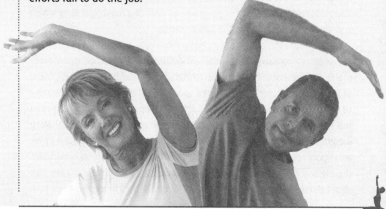

Low Estrogen Promotes
Weight Gain in Women

Menopause causes a large <u>decrease</u> in *estrogens* and *progesterone* with a corresponding <u>increase</u> in total and abdominal **obesity.** Several studies show a reduction in abdominal obesity in women in response to estrogen replacement therapy.[74,83]

Analogous to the way *testosterone* reduces male abdominal fat mass, *estrogen* in females reduces *lipoprotein lipase* activity in abdominal adipocytes. *Lipoprotein lipase* converts circulating triglycerides into *free fatty acids* that are readily stored in adipocytes (fat cells).

The control of *lipoprotein lipase* is very complex and involves several hormones. In women, **cortisol,**[96-98] **testosterone,**[99,100] and **insulin**[101] promote lipid accumulation in adipocytes by <u>increasing</u> *lipoprotein lipase* activity, whereas **growth hormone** and **estrogen** <u>decrease</u> lipoprotein lipase (and thus facilitate abdominal weight loss).[12,100,102,103]

Conventional estrogen drugs list side effects that include **weight gain.** One reason is that until recently the most commonly prescribed estrogen and combination estrogen/progestin drugs were **Premarin®** and **Prempro®,** patented compounds that are not identical to the estrogen and progesterone naturally produced in a woman's body. The dose of these drugs was seldom individualized, so women often received too much (or too little) of these hormones for their particular needs.

With the advent of *bioidentical* estrogen drugs that are individually dosed, women whose blood tests reveal <u>low</u> estrogen (and/or progesterone) can precisely *restore* estrogen and progesterone levels to a range that may induce a reduction in abdominal fat mass, along with other benefits.

Natural estrogen compounds are available by prescription from compounding pharmacists. These types of estrogen are *bioidentical* — the hormones are chemically the same as the natural estrogen produced in a woman's body. The types of estrogens commonly used in bioidentical hormone replacement therapy are *estradiol* and *estriol.*

Bioidentical estrogen drugs are prepared using different percentages of estriol and estradiol compounded into a **topical cream.** The most popular compounded bioidentical estrogen used today is bi-estrogen or **bi-est.** It is prescribed as a **topical cream** that may consist of 80% estriol and 20% estradiol, or a percentage ratio individualized to the patient's need. Based on a women's estradiol **blood test** reading, and the body composition changes that occur, the dose of estradiol and estriol in bi-est may be increased or decreased.

An individualized approach to bioidentical hormone restoration is best. A woman will need to carefully monitor and assess her individual responses and report them to her prescribing physician so that adjustments can be made to her hormone regimen. In general, experts in the field of bioidentical hormone restoration suggest that most women feel their best when *estradiol* **blood levels** are in the range of **90–250** pg/mL, a range of estradiol that is common during the majority of the menstrual cycle for most healthy young women.

In addition to natural estrogen, natural ***progesterone*** is an important hormone for women. Natural progesterone cream or ointment is available as a compounded prescription or OTC (over-the-counter) product. The benefit of using a topical product over an oral form is that the topical form avoids the "first pass" effect of metabolism through the liver, and therefore the dosage is lower (than oral forms).

Progestins such as Provera® are not natural progesterone. Provera® is a type of chemical that bears some similarity to natural progesterone but is chemically distinct. Natural progesterone is believed to be a safer option for women seeking hormone restoration.

There are studies showing increased risks of certain cancers in response to estrogen drug therapy and higher estrogen levels.[104,105] Many of these studies used Premarin® or Prempro®, drugs that many women today avoid because of the lethal risks that were revealed. In response to concerns about estrogen and cancer, *Life Extension*® compiled an article titled **"Is Fear of Cancer a Reason to Be Deprived of Hormones?"** This article discusses healthy dietary and lifestyle alterations that have been shown to substantially reduce the risk of estrogen-induced cancers. Anyone contemplating estrogen replacement therapy should review this article at **www.lef.org/estrogen**. Refer to the sidebar *How To Safely Restore Youthful Hormone Levels In Aging Females on page* 48 for specific information about how your doctor can prescribe bioidentical female hormones and blood levels of these hormones to strive for.

Some obese women have elevated *testosterone* levels.[106,107] Studies show that certain subgroups of obese women (for example, obese women suffering from *polycystic ovary syndrome* [PCOS], characterized by excess visceral body fat, insulin resistance, and high levels of testosterone) can improve metabolic profiles, reduce visceral fat accumulation, and reduce testosterone levels with a combination of *metformin* and low-dose *flutamide,* a specific anti-androgen drug available by prescription.[108,109] For example, a study of 40 obese women suffering from elevated testosterone levels and insulin resistance treated with metformin (850 mg twice daily) and flutamide (250 mg twice daily) showed <u>decreased</u> visceral fat, total cholesterol, and low-density lipoprotein (LDL), and reduced excess testosterone concentrations.[110] If a blood test reveals excess free testosterone in the presence of excess visceral fat in a woman, consider prescribing 250 mg of flutamide twice daily with concomitant metformin treatment in addition to a low-calorie diet and physical exercise.

Weight Loss May Be Impossible if Thyroid Hormone Levels Are Insufficient

The *thyroid gland* secretes hormones involved in cellular energy expenditure. When a person restricts their calorie intake (i.e., goes on a diet), there is often a decrease in metabolically active thyroid hormones that causes the body's fat-burning processes to slow down.

One reason people put on weight is that aging impairs their ability to efficiently utilize carbohydrates and fats. One cause of impaired carbohydrate and lipid metabolism is overt hypothyroidism or sub-clinical thyroid deficiency. Some physicians believe that sub-clinical thyroid deficiency can contribute to unwanted weight gain with advancing age.[111,112]

To give you an idea of how profoundly the thyroid gland dictates body weight, when the thyroid produces too much thyroid hormone, the most common clinical symptom is significant weight loss. The name for the disease caused by an overactive thyroid gland is hyperthyroidism, and in 76%–83% of cases, a patient's first complaint to their physician is about how much weight they have been losing.

In the 1960s and 1970s, the connection between hypothyroidism and weight gain caused some people to assume they could speed up their metabolism and lose weight by using supplemental thyroid hormones. This led to an abuse of thyroid hormone as people created an artificial state of excess thyroid hormone. Hyperthyroidism can cause weight loss as well as irregular heartbeats, sweating, and tremors. Although people taking supplemental thyroid hormones in these studies may have lost weight, they were losing lean muscle mass in addition to excess body fat.[113]

Today we understand that when calorie intake is drastically lowered, the activity of an enzyme called *5'-monodeiodinase* is reduced. *5'-monodeiodinase* is necessary to convert the thyroid

(Continued on page 44)

How to Safely Restore Youthful Testosterone in Aging Men

The use of topical testosterone creams has skyrocketed over the past decade in response to a plethora of positive research findings and endorsements from prominent physician-scientists. While balancing sex hormones in women is challenging, it is quite easy to achieve optimal hormone balance in aging men. What follows is a simple protocol to optimize a male's free testosterone level:

1. Have your blood tested for **free testosterone, estradiol,** and **PSA,** along with complete blood counts and blood chemistries. These blood tests are all included in the comprehensive *Life Extension®* **Male Blood Test Panel**.

2. If these blood test results reveal **free testosterone** below 20 pg/mL and you exhibit signs/ symptoms of low testosterone (e.g. fatigue, loss of libido, abdominal body fat, irritable mood, anxiety) consider asking your doctor to prescribe natural testosterone cream.

3. To obtain **natural testosterone cream** at the <u>lowest</u> price, ask your doctor to consider writing a prescription for <u>compounded</u> natural testosterone cream. A sample prescription for a two-month supply of natural testosterone cream is shown on the next page.

4. The approximate testosterone dose is based on the blood test results and body mass. After 45–60 days, have your blood retested to be prescribed a more precise testosterone dose. Each individual varies slightly based on their rate of absorption and internal metabolism. These blood tests also help rule out prostate cancer, guard against excess red blood cell production and excess estradiol conversion, and ensure that liver enzymes are in normal ranges. Digital rectal exams can further help screen for clinically palpable nodules in the prostate . Testosterone is contraindicated in men with existing prostate cancer.[94] Please note that published scientific literature shows that testosterone does not cause prostate cancer.[95]

5. If your blood **estradiol** level is over **30** pg/mL and you exhibit signs/ symptoms of excess estrogen (e.g. gynecomastia, excess abdominal fat), ask your doctor to consider prescribing a very low-dose aromatase-inhibiting drug such as 0.5 mg of Arimidex® twice a week. This will

usually bring estradiol into the optimal range of **20–30** pg/mL. Do not reduce estradiol below **20** pg/mL as this may interfere with the ability of testosterone to induce abdominal fat loss.

You should have your blood tested ahead of time with your results in hand so your doctor can properly prescribe testosterone during your first visit. You can order the **Male Panel Test** that includes all these blood tests and more by calling **1-800-208-3444.**

Compounded testosterone cream can be obtained for as little as **$40** for a 60-day supply, as opposed to around **$450** for a 60-day supply of conventional testosterone gels.

Your Doctor's Name_____ DEA#_____
Your Doctor's Address_____
Your Doctor's Phone Number_____
Patient's Name_____ Age_____
Address_____Date_____

TESTOSTERONE 100 *mg/mL pump*
Apply 1 *mL (100 mg) daily or as directed*
FILL # 2-month supply (60 mL)

Refill____3____times _____
(Signature)

hormone T4 into T3. When *5'-monodeiodinase* levels are reduced, the levels of T3 drop.[114-117] T3 is the stronger form of thyroid hormone.

Decreased T3 levels can be directly replaced. Studies showed that direct T3 supplementation by dieters was connected with muscle wasting.[118,119] During fasting, administration of large doses of T3 caused even more severe muscle wasting.[120]

More recent studies suggest that using very low doses of replacement thyroid hormone during dieting, once the body has switched over from carbohydrate burning to fat burning, may not be associated with muscle breakdown.[119-121]

Optimizing Thyroid Hormones

While studies show that thyroid supplementation promotes weight loss in some people, it should only be used when there is evidence of a documented thyroid hormone *deficiency,* either in the form of decreased secretion from the thyroid gland or decreased conversion of T4 to the metabolically active T3 in the peripheral tissues. Many people's metabolic rate decreases in response to dieting, as their body attempts to conserve body mass.

That means a person with normal thyroid status before dieting may become thyroid-*deficient* because of the reduced intake of calories. This may occur when drugs like **metformin** or natural products are used to suppress appetite. For optimal fat-loss effects, a person may be prescribed small doses of Cytomel® (a prescription form of T3) if their T3 levels are not in the upper one-third range of normal, or if consuming fewer calories results in a reduction of T3 levels.

There are several blood tests used to assess thyroid function. If any of these tests indicate a documented thyroid deficiency, consider asking your doctor to prescribe the appropriate dose of the drug Cytomel® (T3) or Armour® desiccated thyroid to bring your thyroid level into the normal range.

If a blood test shows an increase in *thyroid-stimulating hormone* (TSH), this means that the pituitary gland is over-secreting a hormone to stimulate thyroid function because of an apparent thyroid deficiency. The normal range for TSH can be as wide as 0.2–5.5 mIU/mL. However, if TSH levels are above **2.0 and you have signs/symptoms of thyroid deficiency (e.g. coarse hair and skin, fatigue, difficulty with focus and concentration, elevation in serum cholesterol levels like LDL, unwanted weight gain),** this suggests that you may be hypothyroid and could benefit from Cytomel® or Armour® drug therapy. Remember, the higher the TSH blood level, the more likely you are to be thyroid-deficient.

T4 (or free *thyroxine*) tests the biologically available hormone being secreted by the thyroid gland. If T4 is deficient, most doctors prescribe Synthroid®, which is a synthetic T4 hormone. We recommend Cytomel® (T3) or Armour® desiccated thyroid instead of Synthroid® (T4) because T3 is the metabolically active form of thyroid that aids in thermogenesis (body fat burning).[124] When evaluating T4 blood test results, optimal levels for males seeking to lose weight should be in a range of 8.5–10.5 mcg/dL. Females under age 60 seeking to lose weight should be in the range of 9–11 mcg/dL. Women older than 60 years should be in the range of 8.5–10.7 mcg/dL. If there is too much T4, this is a sign of hyperthyroidism that should receive immediate medical treatment.

Measuring the amount of T3 is one way of ascertaining how much metabolically active thyroid hormone is available to the tissues. The normal free T3 range is 2.3–4.4 pg/mL. But for losing weight, you might want a range of 3.4–4.4 pg/mL. If your blood levels are below this, Cytomel® drug therapy should be considered. Some patients are started with 12.5 mcg of Cytomel® twice a day. The dose can be increased if blood T3 levels do not return to a normal range or if symptoms of thyroid deficiency persist. If T3 levels are above normal, this can indicate an overdose of drugs like Synthroid® or Cytomel®, or hyperthyroidism.

It should be emphasized that thyroid hormone must NEVER be abused to facilitate weight loss in individuals with normal thyroid function. Human clinical studies show that when thyroid hormone is given in the absence of thyroid insufficiency, muscle tissue is depleted.[113,118,120] The purpose of testing your thyroid hormone status is to ensure they are in the *optimal* range (upper one-third of the normal reference range for T3).

Suppressing Obesity-Inducing Inflammatory Factors

In recent years, *C-reactive protein* (CRP) has emerged as a reliable marker of many age-related diseases that have a hidden inflammatory component, such as heart disease and cancer. However, scientists are now realizing that CRP may also play a more direct role in disease by contributing to the growing obesity epidemic.

In a recent breakthrough, scientists from the University of Pittsburgh have discovered that CRP interacts directly with a key hormone in the body called **leptin**, which signals satiety as well as promotes the breakdown of fat.[125] Researchers have concluded that by binding to leptin, CRP blocks leptin's ability to pass through the blood-brain barrier to reach the hypothalamus and turn off chronic hunger signals, effectively interfering with leptin's ability to regulate body weight. These exciting results reveal the importance of controlling CRP levels as part of a successful weight-management strategy.

Indeed, studies using the dietary supplement *Irvingia gabonensis* have shown a dramatic reduction in weight accompanied by a marked decline in CRP levels.[126-128] Medications such as **orlistat, metformin,** and medications (like acarbose) that inhibit carbohydrate-digesting enzymes can also reduce CRP.[129,130] There are several **nutritional approaches** that offer a safe and effective means of reducing CRP levels:

• A combination of **vitamins C and E** can help to fight inflammation. A recent placebo-controlled study in 19 overweight subjects found that this antioxidant combination reduced CRP levels by 32% compared with an increase of 50% in the placebo group.[131]

• Consuming a diet rich in **omega-3 fatty acids** has been shown to reduce CRP levels.[132] In the Greek ATTICA Study of over 3,000 men and women, there was a 20% reduction of CRP in participants who most closely adhered to a traditional Mediterranean diet.[133]

• Increasing **soluble fiber** intake successfully reduces inflammation, achieving up to a 28% reduction in CRP levels in overweight individuals.[134] Beta-glucans are an excellent soluble dietary fiber that helps lower CRP levels.[135]

• **Niacin** at a dose of 1,000 mg (which should be used with medical supervision) has been shown to reduce CRP levels by 15%.[136]

• **Vitamin D** is also gaining recognition as a crucial modulator of inflammation. A University of London study demonstrated a 23% reduction in CRP levels following vitamin D supplementation.[137]

• Researchers have found that **vitamin K** status and intake also affect levels of CRP. In an analysis of the Framingham Offspring Study of 1,381 subjects with a mean body mass index of 28.1 (classified as overweight), higher levels of vitamin K status and intake (measured both by vitamin K plasma concentration and intake of the vitamin) were associated with lower levels of CRP.[138]

- **Curcumin**, the active ingredient in the curry spice, turmeric, has been used for centuries as a topical anti-inflammatory in India. Experimental studies confirm that it reverses the threat that elevated CRP levels pose to human endothelial cells.[139,140]

- **Flavonoid antioxidants** found in **tea extracts** and **red wine** can also reduce inflammation. In experimental studies, resveratrol and quercetin, found in red wine, have been shown to suppress the expression of CRP in a dose-dependent manner.[141] In addition, a human study of purified theaflavin extracts (found in black tea) produced a dramatic reduction in disease-causing mediators of inflammation, including CRP.[142]

Restoring Insulin Sensitivity and Further Reducing Postprandial Triglycerides

Metformin, an *oral hypoglycemic* drug that helps lower blood sugar levels in people with type 2 diabetes, has some interesting and beneficial side effects when it comes to weight loss.

Recognizing that metformin-treated diabetics often lose weight, and believing that the drug might reduce patients' food intake, researchers at the St. Louis University Medical Center explored possible mechanisms for this effect in 1998.[143] Twelve obese women with type 2 diabetes who were on no medication were randomly assigned to receive oral metformin (850 mg or 1,700 mg) or a placebo at 8 a.m. for three days. After a six-hour fast on the third day, subjects were given a "meal test" at 2 p.m., at which they were offered sandwich canapés. Just before, the meal subjects rated their hunger on a standard scale, and researchers then recorded the number of sandwiches the subjects ate in three consecutive 10-minute periods. Subjects who had taken metformin at either dose had significantly *decreased* calorie intake compared with placebo recipients, with the higher dose producing the most marked effect. Metformin-treated subjects also rated their hunger as lower, with the 1,700 mg/day dose producing the greatest decrease.

The researchers then studied 48 similar obese diabetic women who had not lost weight using diet alone. These subjects were given a 1,200-calorie diet and were then started on metformin (850 mg) or a placebo twice daily for 24 weeks. The metformin-treated patients lost weight continuously throughout the treatment period, with a mean maximum weight loss **17.6 pounds greater** than the placebo group. The metformin recipients also had lower fasting blood glucose levels as well as lower levels of the hemoglobin A1C molecule that

(Continued on page 50)

How To Safely Restore Youthful Hormone Levels In Aging Females

Most practitioners use the level of **estradiol** in women's blood, along with an assessment of the patient's symptoms to prescribe the initial dose of bioidentical estrogen. The **estradiol** blood level must be considered in context to the other hormones such as **progesterone.** Looking at the **estradiol** blood level alone as a target is somewhat effective but not entirely comprehensive.

Here is an example of how estradiol reading is commonly used as an approximation. In menopause, a woman typically has an estradiol blood level of **0–19** pg/mL. If with compounded **bi-est** (estriol and estradiol) cream, the blood estradiol level goes up to **100** pg/mL, for example, then you know that the **bi-est** is being absorbed and has increased your estradiol level. Your doctor may then assume that the other estrogens also went up. If your menopausal symptoms have resolved, you are losing abdominal fat mass and are happy, most practitioners would stop there and continue you on the dosage you have been using and do periodic follow-up.

If, however, you are still having symptoms of estrogen deficiency, your doctor can increase the bi-est dose or order additional tests such as the **total estrogen** blood test and/or a **urinary estrogen** test to get a better handle on the other estrogens and proceed from there. A typical starting dose for bi-est topical cream prescription might read as shown on the next page.

The dose can be <u>increased</u> when severe symptoms of estrogen deficiency are present.

Any woman with an intact uterus must also be prescribed natural progesterone (not synthetic progestin drugs like Provera®) in a dose that achieves a youthful balance. Natural progesterone produces many benefits when properly balanced with estrogen. A typical twice-daily dose is one-quarter teaspoon of a 2.5% OTC natural progesterone cream applied to a different part of the body twice each day. Progesterone can help the skin appear younger, and many women apply it on certain days to their facial skin. It can also be applied to the breasts and inner thighs. Suggested dosing is as follows:

• **Premenstrual and perimenopausal women**: ¼ tsp. twice daily starting on day 12 of the menstrual cycle continuing up to day 28.

• **Menopausal women**: ¼ tsp. twice daily for 21 days followed by 7 days off.

The dose can be adjusted up or down depending on the symptoms and response.

A typical dose for prescription natural progesterone cream will resemble the second graphic shown below.

A blood level target to strive for in aging women might be:

Estradiol	**90–250 pg/mL**
Progesterone	**2.0–6.0 ng/mL**
Free testosterone	**1.0–2.2 pg/mL**

Remember that too much **free testosterone** in an aging woman induces abdominal weight gain, as does a *deficiency* of **estradiol.** Progesterone may be weight neutral, though some complementary practitioners claim it helps facilitate weight loss. Some doctors seek to increase progesterone levels up to **15** ng/mL.

The objective is to achieve a more youthful sex hormone balance not only to induce abdominal fat loss, but also to improve your overall state of health and well-being. The use of estrogen drugs is contraindicated in women with existing estrogen-receptor positive cancer.

Your Doctor's Name_____DEA#_____
Your Doctor's Address_____
Your Doctor's Phone Number_____
Patient's Name_____Age_____
Address_____Date_____

Bi-est: 0.5 mg estradiol / 2.0 mg estriol per mL
  Apply 1 mL topically every day
  #60 mL

Refill_____times _____(Signature)_____

Your Doctor's Name_____DEA#_____
Your Doctor's Address_____
Your Doctor's Phone Number_____
Patient's Name_____Age_____
Address_____Date_____

  PROGESTERONE cream 50 mg/mL
  Directions: Apply 1 mL (pump) topically
  twice daily or at bedtime) days 1-25
  Dispense: 1 or 2 month supply

Refill_____times _____(Signature)_____

is a marker of chronic blood sugar levels. The authors of this study concluded *"metformin decreases calorie intake in a dose-dependent manner and leads to a reduction in body weight in non-insulin dependent diabetic patients with obesity."*[143]

Metformin's health benefits now appear to extend beyond simple weight loss. Other studies are showing that it can beneficially affect a variety of other parameters that are disturbed by obesity. A group of Turkish researchers, writing in *Internal Medicine* in 2008, demonstrated that, in addition to weight loss, metformin-treated obese subjects had highly significant decreases in hypertension, disruptions of lipid profiles, and fasting blood sugar levels compared with placebo-treated subjects. These researchers ended their report with the statement that *"metformin treatment should be initiated in patients in their fifties with excess weight."*[144] While that may be a bit over-enthusiastic, it does highlight the excitement generated by this drug.

A Mexican research group has made similar findings with greater precision. They treated 60 obese patients with metabolic syndrome (a constellation of findings related to obesity and its consequences), giving them metformin 850 mg/day or a placebo, along with dietary counseling for all patients. They followed the patients for one year, tracking vital indicators of obesity-related cardiovascular health such as BMI, waist circumference, blood pressure, lipid profiles, blood sugar, and markers of the oxidant stress and inflammation that are cardinal features of the metabolic syndrome. Both groups lost weight and had improved blood pressure during the study, but patients taking metformin also had reductions in total cholesterol, markers of oxidation and CRP, a critical marker of inflammation related to vascular health. Perhaps most impressively, treated patients also had significant reductions in their *intima-media thickness* (IMT), which is a direct measure of blood vessel health reflecting the vessels' actual reaction to metabolic risk factors. Not surprisingly these researchers concluded that *"metformin has a considerable beneficial effect on nitroxidation, endothelial function and IMT in patients with metabolic syndrome."*[145]

Metformin has been used by healthy anti-aging enthusiasts since the early 1990s. Its ability to reduce glucose and insulin levels have led some to postulate that metformin may mimic some of the beneficial effects of *caloric restriction.* There are relatively few contraindications for prescribing metformin. Our only concern vis-à-vis this comprehensive weight-loss protocol we are proposing regards hyper-responders to the *alpha-glucosidase* and *alpha-amylase inhibitors* who also overly respond to *metformin.* There is a theoretical risk of inducing a state of *hypoglycemia* when all <u>three</u> agents are combined. In the real world setting, however, most overweight and obese patients will already suffer from some degree of glucose impairment and should benefit greatly from all three of these treatment modalities. A safe starting dose of metformin would be 250 mg twice a day before a meal. If glucose levels are not overly suppressed, the metformin dose can be increased to as high as 850 mg two or even three times a day before meals.

An undesirable side effect of metformin for men is that it can <u>reduce</u> *testosterone* levels.[146] As mentioned earlier, <u>low</u> testosterone predisposes aging men to abdominal obesity. This may be why metformin has not always produced significant weight loss in clinical studies. Men who are prescribed testosterone replacement therapy can readily overcome this side effect if **blood tests** reveal that the prescribed dose of testosterone is not increasing free testosterone blood levels to the optimal **20–25** pg/mL range. All the prescribing doctor has to do is slightly increase the testosterone dose to overcome the testosterone-reducing effect of the metformin.

Optimal Blood Ranges to Facilitate Weight Loss

There are a variety of **blood tests** that can direct what drugs, hormones, and nutrients a doctor may prescribe for you to correct underlying hormonal and metabolic disorders and facilitate weight loss.

An obese individual will often exhibit dangerously high levels of *C-reactive protein.* Not only is this associated with increased vascular disease, dementia, and cancer risk, but it also can preclude weight loss by binding to leptin and creating a state of *leptin resistance.*[125,147-149] Leptin is a satiety hormone that also helps promote the breakdown of triglycerides in adipocytes.[150-152] Most of the drugs suggested in this protocol will induce a significant <u>reduction</u> in *C-reactive protein* blood levels. For men, ideal C-reactive protein is below **0.55** mg/L. Women should be below **1.55** mg/L of blood.

We have learned to accept any reading of fasting *glucose* under **100** mg/dL of blood as acceptable. The reality is that any increase of fasting glucose over **85** mg/dL incrementally increases heart attack risk and probably contributes to unwanted fat accumulation. Ideal fasting glucose is probably in the range of **72–74** mg/dL, but it will be challenging to achieve these levels in overweight and obese individuals even when all the medications suggested in this protocol are concomitantly prescribed.

(Continued on page 54)

Tying It All Together

Overweight and obese individuals are likely to suffer from postprandial disorders that prevent sustainable fat loss. Young healthy humans can often ingest high-calorie meals without accumulating surplus body fat. Young bodies respond with an immediate surge of insulin that precisely converts ingested calories to energy with minimal fat storage. They have abundant functioning insulin receptors capable of optimally regulating how they metabolize their food. Hormones that regulate fat storage are primed to keep young bodies slender.

Normal aging severely disrupts these healthy metabolic patterns, often necessitating aggressive medical interventions. **Blood test** results help show you the degree of metabolic disturbance you may manifest if on a blood test report your fasting triglycerides are far above **60–80** mg/dL and fasting glucose hovers around or greater than **100** mg/dL.

What has become accepted as "normal" blood test findings (within the "reference range") are really an indicator of how widespread metabolic disorders have become in modern societies. An overweight or obese individual with fasting glucose around **100** mg/dL almost always has dangerously high fasting insulin levels. While this surplus insulin may temporarily keep glucose at barely acceptable levels, insulin resistance disrupts normal metabolic processes and contributes to excess storage of body fat. For long-term weight loss to occur, it is critical to enhance insulin sensitivity and purge the excess levels of fats (mainly trlglycerides) and glucose that chronically saturate an overweight individual's bloodstream.

We therefore recommend the following pharmaceutical interventions for the first 60–90 days (or longer in certain patients):

1. **Orlistat**, **120 mg**, can be taken three times a day before each meal to inhibit the lipase enzyme. This will result in a rapid reduction of triglycerides and chronic inflammatory markers with a partial reversal of insulin resistance syndrome.

2. After two days, the drug **acarbose**, **50 mg** three times a day before meals, can be introduced to inhibit the *alpha-glucosidase* enzyme.

3. Patients presenting indications of metabolic syndrome, pre-diabetes, or frank type 2 diabetes should be considered for **metformin** therapy. Initial dose should be 250 mg with the two largest meals of the day.

The dose may be increased to 850 mg taken with each meal (up to 2,550 mg/day). Metformin functions via multiple mechanisms to improve a patient's metabolic profile while helping to suppress appetite.

4. **Men** with signs/symptoms of hypogonadism (e.g., low libido, low muscle mass, abdominal obesity, fatigue, anxiety, irritability) and free **testosterone** levels below optimal ranges of 20 pg/mL of blood can be prescribed a **compounded testosterone cream** to increase their free testosterone to optimal levels (20–25 pg/mL of blood). Low testosterone predisposes men to abdominal obesity. Men with existing prostate cancer should not be prescribed testosterone. Estradiol levels in men should be maintained in the range of 20–30 pg/mL of blood based upon the available scientific evidence at the time of this writing.

5. **Women** with signs/ symptoms of insufficient estrogen and **estradiol** levels below 90 pg/mL of blood can be prescribed a compounded **bio-identical estriol/estradiol cream** to increase their estradiol blood reading to over 90 pg/mL of blood. Women deficient in estrogen are predisposed to abdominal fat accumulation. Women with existing estrogen receptor positive cancers should not be prescribed estrogen drugs. All women with an intact uterus should be prescribed natural progesterone and most will benefit by restoring progesterone blood levels to the youthful range. Women with excess free testosterone can be prescribed metformin and flutamide as discussed earlier.

6. **Thyroid** status can be assessed with blood tests and patients' free T3 level should be kept in the upper one-third range of normal, but it should never be increased to above the upper range of normal. Ensuring compliance is critical to achieve meaningful weight loss.

The standard reference range for fasting triglycerides extends up to **149** mg/dL of blood, but any number above **80** mg/dL is probably too high. To protect against vascular disease, triglyceride levels should be suppressed far <u>below</u> **100** mg/dL. To treat the *postprandial lipemia* that has been identified as a probable cause of obesity, suppressing triglyceride levels <u>below</u> **60** mg/dL of blood would be ideal, though most overweight individuals will be challenged to achieve these levels. Scientists have identified a phenomenon known as *postprandial hypertriglyceridemia,* in which triglyceride levels remain high after a meal. This represents a significant independent risk factor for vascular disease. Have your blood tested two to three hours after you have ingested a typical meal. A person with acceptable *fasting* triglycerides might demonstrate higher than desirable (greater than 133 mg/dL) *postprandial* triglycerides. The medications and nutrients suggested in this protocol should sharply reduce triglyceride levels and help purge the bloodstream of chronic postprandial lipemia that contributes to surplus body fat stores.

The reference range for thyroid hormone tests can cause those with less than optimal thyroid hormone levels to be diagnosed as "normal." Make sure your TSH is <u>below</u> **2.00** mIU/mL of blood and *free* T3 is in the **upper one-third** of the standard reference range.

For many aging men, a *free testosterone* blood reading of **20–25** pg/mL appears to be optimal, while estradiol levels should be kept at **20–30** pg/mL of blood at the time of this writing, based upon the existing scientific evidence.

The optimal blood level of *estradiol* in aging women varies considerably. An estradiol target to attain using bioidentical estrogens is **90–250** pg/mL. If this range helps facilitate abdominal fat loss, then it may be ideal for you. If you are ever prescribed estrogen, it is imperative that you follow the cancer risk-reduction program that can be accessed by logging on to **www.lef.org/estrogen**. Remember that in females, excess free testosterone may contribute to abdominal obesity. So if a blood test reveals above range testosterone, ask your doctor to prescribe the appropriate medications (metformin and/or flutamide).

Managing "Unrealistic" Weight-Loss Expectations

Clinical studies document that overweight and obese subjects have unrealistic expectations about the rapidity and amount of body fat loss that will occur in response to weight-loss drugs.[153]

For many, if <u>immediate</u> fat-loss results do not occur, they abandon the program, even though they've been repeatedly told that weight loss is a gradual process. Regrettably, the desire for major cosmetic weight loss and the lack of understanding of the medical benefits derived from modest body fat reduction can conspire to derail the best-laid scientific protocols.

A key element to short- and long-term success is to understand the importance of continuous compliance.

Addressing psychological issues such as *emotional eating* are important considerations. Drugs like Wellbutrin® and Adderall® have been shown to induce weight loss, but can cause psychological disturbances.[154-156] Likewise, the drug *sibutramine* (Meridia®) has demonstrated potent weight-loss properties.[157,158] Sibutramine reduces the reuptake of serotonin (by 54%), norepinephrine (by 73%), and dopamine (by 16%), thereby increasing the levels of these transmitters in the brain and helping to enhance early satiety.[159]

As explained earlier, those with emotional eating issues may benefit from a supplement designed to deliver greater amounts of tryptophan into the brain for conversion to serotonin.

Summary: Is All of This Too Complicated?

You may be wondering if this multi-pronged approach to optimally induce immediate and sustainable weight loss is too complicated and expensive.

Fortunately, *Life Extension®* offers a comprehensive Male or Female Weight Loss Blood Test Panel at very **low** prices. (For information, please visit **www.lef.org/bloodtest**, or call **1-800-208-3444**.) Many of the drugs can be obtained in very low-cost generic or compounded form. There are also nutritional supplements that can be substituted for some of the medications. So the cost of implementing this program is affordable for most individuals.

As far as the complexities of this protocol, remember that an estimated 300,000 Americans die each year due to obesity.[160] Looking at this data, it becomes rapidly apparent that the metabolic dysfunction displayed outwardly in the form of **excess body fat** is by far the <u>leading</u> killer. Be it stroke, heart attack, dementia, or cancer, the more *overweight* you are, the <u>greater</u> the likelihood you will be stricken by these lethal diseases.

For the past 50 years, a wide variety of methods have been attempted to overcome the worsening obesity epidemic. Yet, there are more overweight Americans now than ever before. Until a magic bullet is discovered, the only way to achieve optimal weight control for many people may be to follow most, if not all, of the suggestions you have just read.

If you have any questions on the scientific content of this book, please call a Life Extension Health Advisor at 1-866-820-8083.

References:
1. *Curr Hypertens Rep.* 2008 Feb;10(1):32-8.
2. *Lancet.* 2005 Apr 16;365(9468):1415-28.
3. *Diabetes.* 1996 Jul;45(Suppl 3):S59-61.
4. *J Nutr Biochem.* 2008 Aug;19(8):491-504.
5. *Am J Physiol Heart Circ Physiol.* 2007 Feb;292(2):H904-11.
6. *Nutr Rev.* 2007 Dec;65(12 Pt 2):S253-9.
7. *Prev Med.* 2006 May;42(5):336-42.
8. *Acta Physiol* Scand. 2005 Aug;184(4):285-93.
9. *Curr Atheroscler Rep.* 2004 Nov;6(6):424-31.
10. *Postgrad Med J.* 1969 September; 45(527): 602–607.
11. *JAMA.* 2002 Dec 4;288(21):2709-16.
12. *Metab Syndr Relat Disord.* 2007 Dec;5(4):291-6.
13. *Med Sci* (Paris). 2005 Dec;21 Spec No10-8.
14. *Metab Syndr Relat Disord.* 2008 Winter;6(4):299-304.
15. *Obes Rev.* 2009 Mar;10(Suppl 1):24-33.
16. http://www.nlm.nih.gov/medlineplus/druginfo/meds/a601244.html
17. *Am J Clin Nutr.* 2007 Jun;85(6):1511-20.
18. *Clin Ther.* 2005;27(Suppl B):S42-56.
19. http://www.sciencedirect.com/science?_ob=ArticleURL&_udi=B83WG-4S1C3S2-6&_user=10&_rdoc=1&_fmt=&_orig=search&_sort=d&view=c&_acct=C000050221&_version=1&_urlVersion=0&_userid=10&md5=36aa01bb7107426818b8e8747f3cf0aa
20. *Stroke.* 2004 May;35(5):1073-8.
21. *Eur Heart J.* 2004 Jan;25(1):10-6.
22. *Int J Cardiol.* 2006 Feb 8;107(1):11-20.
23. Aronson JK. *Meyler's Side Effects of Endocrine and Metabolic Drugs.* New York, NY: Elsevier Science; 2008:361.
24. *Curr Diabetes Rev.* 2008 Nov;4(4):340-56.
25. *Nutrition.* 2005 Jul-Aug;21(7-8):848-54.
26. *Altern Med Rev.* 2004 Mar;9(1):63-9.
27. http://www.cspinet.org/new/sugar_limit.html
28. *Journal of Nutrition* 2001; 131: 796-799.
29. "A Pilot Study of the Effects of L-A/Cr: A Novel Combination of L-Arabinose and a Patented Chromium Supplement on Serum Glucose Levels After Sucrose Challenges," Gilbert R. Kaats, Ph.D., FACN; Harry Preuss, MD, MACN; Joel E. Michalek, Ph.D; Samuel C. Keith, BBA; Patti Keith, BBA; 2009
30. *JAMA.* 2007 Jul 18;298(3):299-308.
31. *J Am Diet Assoc.* 1998 Oct;98(10 Suppl 2):S23-6.
32. *Drugs Today* (Barc). 1999 Feb;35(2):139-45.
33. *Prim Care.* 2003 Jun;30(2):427-40.
34. *Obesity* (Silver Spring). 2008 Mar;16(3):623-9.
35. *Drugs.* 2006;66(12):1625-56.
36. *Obes Res.* 2000 Jan;8(1):49-61.
37. *Arq Bras Cardiol.* 2007 Dec;89(6):409-14.
38. *Hormones* (Athens). 2006 Oct;5(4):259-69.
39. *Am J Cardiol.* 2003 Apr 15;91(8):961-4.
40. *Angiology.* 2007 Feb;58(1):26-33.
41. *J Physiol Biochem.* 2009 Sep;65(3):215-23.
42. *Arch Intern Med.* 2010 Jan 25;170(2):136-45

43. *Eat Weight Disord.* 2006 Mar;11(1):e35-41.
44. *Metab Syndr Relat Disord.* 2005;3(2):122-9.
45. *Am J Med.* 1997 Jan;102(1):99-110.
46. *Advances in Therapy.* 1997 Jan 1;14(6):338–47.
47. *Drugs.* 1999;58(Suppl 1):71-3.
48. *Diabetes Care.* 2001 Mar;24(3):489-94.
49. *Biochem Biophys Res Commun.* 2002 Nov 15;298(5):779-84.
50. *Arterioscler Thromb Vasc Biol.* 1995 Dec;15(12):2111-21.
51. *Am J Clin Nutr.* 2006 Dec;84(6):1290-8.
52. *Ir J Med Sci.* 2005 Jan-Mar;174(1):8-20.
53. *Am J Clin Nutr.* 2003 Mar;77(3):605-11.
54. *Curr Opin Lipidol.* 2002 Feb;13(1):33-40.
55. *J Am Coll Nutr.* 2000 Jun;19(3):383-91.
56. *J Nutr.* 2002 Jul;132(7):1879-85.
57. *J Nutr.* 2005 Jun;135(6):1339-42.
58. *J Nutr.* 2004 Apr;134(4):880-5.
59. *Am J Clin Nutr.* 2003 Feb;77(2):300-7.
60. *Am J Clin Nutr.* 2000 Apr;71(4):914-20.
61. *Nutr Metab Cardiovasc Dis.* 2001 Feb;11(1):7-16.
62. *Atherosclerosis.* 2006 Apr;185(2):313-9.
63. *Br J Nutr.* 2005 Apr;93(4):543-7.
64. *Sports Med.* 2006;36(7):547-60.
65. *Arch Intern Med.* 2000 Apr 24;160(8):1177-84.
66. *Am J Cardiol.* 2000 May 1;85(9):1100-5.
67. *Diabetes Care.* 2005 Apr;28(4):844-9.
68. *Metabolism.* 1998 Apr;47(4):371-6.
69. *Diabetologia.* 2006 Mar;49(3):527-37.
70. *Exp Clin Endocrinol Diabetes.* 2005 Feb;113(2):80-4.
71. *Am J Cardiol.* 2004 Jan 1;93(1):31-9.
72. *Atherosclerosis.* 2004 Feb;172(2):375-82.
73. *Chin Med J* (Engl). 2003 Mar;116(3):453-8.
74. *Obes Rev.* 2004 Nov;5(4):197-216.
75. *Eur Heart J.* 2002 May;23(9):706-13.
76. *Circulation.* 2008 Apr 1;117(13):1658-67.
77. *J Endocrinol Invest.* 2006;29(3 Suppl):77-82.
78. http://www.cancer.gov/cancertopics/factsheet/risk/obesity
79. *J Natl Cancer Inst.* 2006 Jul 5;98(13):920-31.
80. *Int J Obes Relat Metab Disord.* 2002 Jun;26(6):747-53.
81. *Curr Urol Rep.* 2007 Nov;8(6):467-71.
82. *Curr Opin Endocrinol Diabetes Obes.* 2007 Jun;14(3):226-34.
83. *Maturitas.* 2008 May 20;60(1):10-8.
84. *J Clin Endocrinol Metab.* 2008 Jan;93(1):139-46.
85. *J Clin Endocrinol Metab.* 1995 Jan;80(1):239-43.
86. *Clin Endocrinol* (Oxf). 2005 Sep;63(3):239-50.
87. *Int J Obes Relat Metab Disord.* 2000 Apr;24(4):485-91.
88. *Obes Res.* 1995 Nov;3(Suppl 4):609S-12S.
89. *J Clin Endocrinol Metab.* 2001 Aug;86(8):3604-10.
90. *Int J Obes Relat Metab Disord.* 1995 Sep;19(9):614-24.
91. *Arterioscler Thromb Vasc Biol.* 1996 Nov;16(11):1383-7.
92. *Neurology.* 2007 Feb 20;68(8):563-8.
93. *Metabolism.* 1997 Feb;46(2):179-85.
94. *J Clin Endocrinol Metab.* 2006 Jun;91(6):1995-2010.
95. *Cancer Epidemiol Biomarkers Prev.* 1996 Aug;5(8):621-5.
96. *Psychosom Med.* 2000 Sep;62(5):623-32.
97. *Metabolism.* 1992 Aug;41(8):882-6.
98. *Metabolism.* 1980 Oct;29(10):980-5.
99. *J Clin Endocrinol Metab.* 1990 Feb;70(2):473-9.
100. *J Clin Invest.* 1988 Sep;82(3):1106-12.
101. *J Clin Invest.* 1982 May;69(5):1119-25.
102. *Am J Obstet Gynecol.* 1998 Jan;178(1 Pt 1):101-7.
103. *J Clin Endocrinol Metab.* 1995 Mar;80(3):936-41.
104. *Am J Epidemiol.* 2008 May 15;167(10):1207-16.
105. *JAMA.* 2008 Mar 5;299(9):1036-45.

106. *J Steroid Biochem Mol Biol*. 2008 Feb;108(3-5):272-80.
107. *Obesity* (Silver Spring). 2009 Jan 29.
108. *J Clin Endocrinol Metab*. 2006 Oct;91(10):3970-80.
109. *Hum Reprod*. 2003 Jan;18(1):57-60.
110. *Clin Endocrinol* (Oxf). 2004 Feb;60(2):241-9.
111. *J Fam Pract*. 1994 Jun;38(6):577-82.
112. *Thyroid*. 1998 Sep;8(9):803-13.
113. Kasper DL, Braunwald E, Hauser SL, Longo DL, Jameson JL. *Harrison's Principles of Internal Medicine*. 16th ed. New York, NY: McGraw-Hill Professional; 2004.
114. *Metabolism*. 1976 Jan;25(1):79-83.
115. *J Clin Endocrinol Metab*. 1977 Oct;45(4):707-13.
116. *J Endocrinol*. 1989 Feb;120(2):337-50.
117. *Int J Obes*. 1990 Mar;14(3):249-58.
118. *N Engl J Med*. 1979 Mar 15;300(11):579-84.
119. *Trans Assoc Am Physicians*. 1978;91:169-79.
120. *Metabolism*. 1975 Oct;24(10):1177-83.
121. *Int J Obes*. 1989;13(4):487-96.
122. *J Clin Endocrinol Metab*. 1996 Mar;81(3):968-76.
123. *Clin Endocrinol* (Oxf). 1984 Oct;21(4):357-67.
124. *Thyroid*. 2008 Feb;18(2):197-203.
125. *Nat Med*. 2006 Apr;12(4):425-32.
126. *Lipids Health Dis*. 2009 Mar 2;8:7.
127. *Lipids Health Dis*. 2005 May 25;4:12.
128. *Lipids Health Dis*. 2008 Nov 13;7:44.
129. *Acta Cardiol*. 2005 Jun;60(3):265-9.
130. *J Clin Endocrinol Metab*. 2003 Oct;88(10):4649-54.
131. *Obesity* (Silver Spring). 2008 Jul;16(7):1573-8.
132. *Horm Metab Res*. 2008 Mar;40(3):199-205.
133. *J Am Coll Cardiol*. 2004 Jul 7;44(1):152-8.
134. *JAMA*. 2003 Jul 23;290(4):502-10.
135. *J Am Coll Nutr*. 2008 Jun;27(3):434-40.
136. *Am J Cardiol*. 2006 Sep 15;98(6):743-5.
137. *QJM*. 2002 Dec;95(12):787-96.
138. *Am J Epidemiol*. 2008 Feb 1;167(3):313-20.
139. *Thromb Res*. 2008;122(1):125-33.
140. *Surgery*. 2005 Aug;138(2):212-22.
141. *J Thromb Haemost*. 2007 Jun;5(6):1309-17.
142. WG0401 protective against generalized inflammation in a human study. Unpublished data, WellGen, Inc.; 2007.
143. *Obes Res*. 1998 Jan;6(1):47-53.
144. *Intern Med*. 2008;47(8):697-703.
145. *Clin Exp Pharmacol* Physiol. 2008 Aug;35(8):895-903.
146. *Obes Res*. 2001 Nov;9(11):662-7.
147. *Curr Hypertens* Rep. 2008 Apr;10(2):131-7.
148. *Front Biosci*. 2007;12:3531-44.
149. *Obesity* (Silver Spring). 2006 Aug;14(Suppl 5):254S-8S.
150. *Endocr J*. 2008 Oct;55(5):827-37.
151. *Exp Biol Med* (Maywood). 2005 Mar;230(3):200-6.
152. *FASEB J*. 2001 Feb;15(2):333-40.
153. *J Consult Clin Psychol*. 2003 Dec;71(6):1084-9.
154. *J Clin Psychopharmacol*. 2006 Aug;26(4):409-13.
155. *Prague Med Rep*. 2005;106(3):291-6.
156. *Clin Ther*. 2006 Feb;28(2):266-79.
157. *Eur J Pharmacol*. 2000 May 26;397(1):93-102.
158. *Int J Obes Relat Metab Disord*. 1998 Aug;22(Suppl 1):S18-28.
159. http://www.fda.gov/cder/foi/label/2006/020632s026lbl.pdf.
160. http://www.cdc.gov/nchs/FASTATS/deaths.htm.
161. *Arch Intern Med*. 2007 May 14;167(9):893-902.
162. *FASEB J*. 2000 Jun;14(9):1132-8.
163. *Obes Surg*. 1993 Nov;3(4):421-4.
164. *Curr Atheroscler Rep*. 2003 Nov;5(6):445-51.
165. *Appl Physiol Nutr Metab*. 2007 Jun;32(3):473-80.

CHAPTER 3

A Multi-Modal Approach to Combat Obesity

A question middle-aged people ask is why they amass so much body fat while eating *less* than when they were younger <u>and</u> thinner. Scientists have identified a number of biological factors to explain age-related weight gain. Yet effective programs to restore youthful body contours remain elusive.

A major impediment to circumventing the *causes* of weight gain is the simple fact that there are so many causes. The encouraging news is that there are <u>more</u> scientifically documented weight-loss compounds to <u>neutralize</u> these *obesity factors* than ever before.

When used in controlled clinical studies, these compounds have demonstrated modest to impressive fat-loss effects. These same benefits are not always duplicated in real world settings. What has yet to be done, until now, is to combine scientifically validated compounds into a ***multi-modal*** program that circumvents *every* known factor involved in excess *age-related* fat storage.

The Age-Related Decrease in Cellular Energy Expenditure

We know that <u>one</u> factor involved in age-related weight gain is a decrease in *resting energy expenditure* at the cellular level. We are not burning fat as energy and instead are storing it in our adipocytes (fat cells). Our bloated outer appearance reflects this *relentless* engorgement of surplus fat into our adipocytes.

Scientists have estimated that the ***decrease*** in energy expenditure with aging may cause **120–190 excess calories** to be stored in the body every day.[2] This translates to an **extra 13–20 pounds** of stored body fat each year.

Based on these data, the restoration of a more **youthful metabolic rate** is <u>one</u> critical factor in inducing weight loss in aging people. Fortunately, a patented **green tea delivery system** has been documented to **significantly enhance weight loss** and **reduce abdominal waist circumference** in humans.

This new *green tea phytosome* delivery system is only <u>one</u> part of a ***multi-modal*** solution to do away with surplus **body fat.**

The Making of a Superior
Green Tea Compound

A number of published studies demonstrate weight-loss effects in response to ingesting green tea or specific tea extracts. A problem identified early on is getting *enough* of green tea's active constituents absorbed into the bloodstream and delivered to cells throughout the body.

The key components responsible for green tea's weight-loss benefits are the *polyphenol* compounds that increase *metabolic energy expenditure* and hence calorie consumption.[3-7] Scientists realized that these *polyphenols* would be more effective if their absorption from the intestinal tract could be *increased* and thus deliver <u>more</u> of the metabolically active agent to the tissues.[8-11]

A group of Italian researchers created biological *complexes* of purified *green tea polyphenols* combined with *phospholipids*. This unique ***green tea phytosome*** was shown to <u>increase</u> the polyphenols' ability to be absorbed after oral ingestion and increase peak plasma levels of the critical green tea polyphenol *epigallocatechin gallate* (EGCG). After oral ingestion of an equal dose of EGCG complexed with phospholipids, the peak plasma level was **138% <u>greater</u>** than for EGCG alone! Furthermore, the total amount of EGCG measured over time was about **three times greater** for the phospholipid complex than for the free form alone![8]

Dramatic Weight Loss!

When this purified ***green tea phytosome*** was tested on human subjects, the weight-loss effects were rapid and substantial. This in-depth multicenter clinical trial involved 100 significantly overweight participants.[8] Half the group received the ***green tea phytosome*** (two **150 mg** tablets daily). Both groups were placed on reduced calorie diets (approximately 1,850 calories/day for men and 1,350 calories/day for women).

After **45** days, the control group lost an average of around **four** pounds. The groups receiving the green tea phytosome supplement dropped an average of 13 pounds — more than **triple** the amount of the control group.

After **90** days, the results were virtually unprecedented! The control group that followed the restricted calorie diet alone lost **9.9** pounds. The ***green tea phytosome***-supplemented group shed a total of **30.1 pounds** — again more than <u>triple</u> the amount of weight loss compared with the control group![8]

Impressive Reduction in Abdominal Circumference

Study subjects in the group receiving the **green tea phytosome** had a **12%** <u>decrease</u> in their *body mass index* (BMI) compared with only **5%** <u>decrease</u> in the diet-alone group.[8]

In the all-important measurement of waist circumference (abdominal girth), there was a **10%** <u>reduction</u> in the **green tea phytosome** group compared with a **5%** <u>reduction</u> in the diet-alone group. Male participants did even better in this category, showing a **14%** <u>reduction</u> in waist circumference compared with a **7%** reduction in the control group.[8]

Green Tea Does More Than Boost Metabolic Rate

As we age, we have a reduced **metabolic capacity** to make use of the fats and sugars we eat throughout the day. The result is that our bloodstreams become chronically *bloated* with artery-clogging and obesity-inducing dietary byproducts.

A proven way to *reverse* the chronic **fat-sugar overload** in our blood is to impede its *absorption* from the digestive tract. While there are drugs that effectively do this, *green tea extracts* have demonstrated promise as inhibitors of fat absorption.[12,13] The ability of green tea to inhibit *absorption* of ingested fat calories may explain some of the observed vascular risk reduction that had been previously ascribed purely to its antioxidant effects.[13]

How Green Tea Inhibits Fat Absorption <u>and</u> Fat Accumulation in Cells

French researchers released a landmark paper demonstrating that a **green tea extract** inhibited the breakdown of fat molecules in the digestive tract that enable these fats to be absorbed from the intestine.[12]

They found that green tea extract could inhibit fat-digesting enzymes in the stomach and small intestine in animal studies, concluding that *"green tea extract exhibiting marked inhibition of digestive lipases is likely to reduce fat digestion in humans."*[12]

Researchers at Rutgers University demonstrated much more recently that these fat-absorption-reducing effects of green tea extracts could inhibit the development of obesity, the metabolic syndrome, and fatty liver disease in mice.[15] Korean researchers last year showed that *green tea extracts* could reduce weight gain in mice by impeding dietary fat absorption and by modulating activity of the gene target PPAR-*gamma*.[16] In another **2008** report, the same team demonstrated that certain *green tea extracts* prevent fat from accumulating inside fat cells.[17]

Reduction of Obesity Factor Blood Markers

This **green tea phytosome** demonstrated still other benefits that help to explain <u>how</u> it induced so much **fat loss** in the human study (described on the previous page).

In the diet-alone control group, total **cholesterol** dropped **10%** and **triglycerides** dropped **20%**. These reductions are expected in response to a reduction in calorie intake.[8] In the **green tea phytosome**-supplemented group, however, total cholesterol dropped **25%** and **triglycerides** dropped **33%**.[8]

An important element involved in successful *weight loss* is to purge excess fat (triglycerides) from the bloodstream. Study subjects taking this **green tea phytosome** significantly reduced their **blood levels** of **triglycerides** (and cholesterol). This may help explain the remarkable reduction of **30.1 pounds** of body weight experienced by those receiving this novel polyphenol compound most aptly named **TeaSlender™ Green Tea Phytosome**.

There has been a veritable explosion of research into how green tea extracts affect every aspect of obesity, from inhibition of fat breakdown and absorption in the digestive tract, to reduction in fat storage within cells, to enhancement of metabolic rate with concomitant increased energy consumption.[3,16-18] All of these benefits indicate an important role for green tea in helping to prevent the deadly *metabolic syndrome,* a constellation of disease risk factors that are often initiated by obesity.[19,20]

How Carbohydrates Induce Weight Gain

The weight-loss effects of blocking dietary fat absorption are not as profound as one might expect. One reason is that in the aging body, **carbohydrates** absorbed into the bloodstream are readily transformed into *triglycerides*, the primary form that fat is stored in the adipocytes.

The aging body develops a resistance to the ability of insulin to transport glucose into the body's energy-producing cells. This excess glucose promotes chronic secretion of **insulin** into the bloodstream *(hyper-insulinemia),* and chronically elevated insulin levels are associated with excess fat storage and degenerative diseases. As excess glucose accumulates in the blood, it is converted by an enzyme *(glycerol-3-phosphate dehydrogenase)* into triglycerides for storage in the adipocytes (fat cells).

Scientists refer to the chronic bloodstream-overload of sugars and fats as *postprandial (*after meal) *disorders*. For significant and sustained fat loss to occur, one should <u>reduce</u> postprandial blood levels of both sugar (glucose) <u>and</u> fat (triglycerides).

Impeding Carbohydrate Absorption

Blocking the breakdown and absorption of carbohydrates are important points of intervention for losing weight. The objective is to target specific *enzymes* in the intestine, *before* calorie-rich carbohydrates enter the circulation.

Researchers at the innovative Integrative Medicine Program at the UCLA School of Medicine have been actively exploring this area, using extracts from the common white kidney bean *(Phaseolus vulgaris)*.[21] The bean extract attains its effect by targeting the *alpha-amylase* starch-digesting enzymes in the intestine.[22] In order to validate this theory, a study was done where 27 obese adults took either a placebo or the **Phaseolus vulgaris** extract.[21] After eight weeks, those taking the white bean extract lost **3.8 pounds** in weight, and **1.5 inches** of abdominal fat. Another important benefit in those taking the **Phaseolus vulgaris** was a **three-fold <u>reduction</u>** in *triglyceride* levels compared with the placebo recipients.

In another human study of *Phaseolus vulgaris*,[23] researchers discovered that those who consumed the most carbohydrates lost the most weight. Those study subjects consuming the highest levels of dietary starch and supplemented with **Phaseolus vulgaris** lost **8.7 pounds** compared with only **1.7 pounds** in the control group. Even more impressive was the **3.3 inches** of belly fat lost in the **Phaseolus vulgaris** group versus only **1.3 inches** in the controls. The conclusions showed that weight loss is attainable with diet modification, exercise, and behavioral interventions and it can be optimized in people with high starch intakes through the addition of **Phaseolus vulgaris**.

In a remarkable double-blind study on 60 overweight volunteers, half the study participants received **445** mg a day of **Phaseolus vulgaris** while the other half were given a placebo.[24] Both groups were placed on a 2,000–2,200/day-calorie, carbohydrate-rich diet. After only **30 days,** those taking **Phaseolus vulgaris** lost **6.5 pounds** of weight and **1.2 inches** in waist size compared with **0.8 pounds** and **0.2 inches** in the placebo group.

These kinds of studies show the futility of trying to lose weight by restricting caloric intake alone, yet demonstrate remarkable effects when just <u>one</u> natural weight loss compound is <u>combined</u> with reductions in food intake.

Targeting the *Alpha-Glucosidase* Enzyme

While inhibiting intestinal *amylase* enzyme activity has demonstrated some fat-loss results, it may be equally important to impede another enzyme needed for carbohydrate absorption called *alpha-glucosidase.*

European researchers working with extracts of several seaweed species found that extracts of the *Fucus vesiculosus* (bladderwrack) caused significant *reductions* in blood glucose eight hours after being given to rabbits.[25] Subsequent research has uncovered a host of health benefits from seaweed extracts, including powerful antioxidant, anti-tumor, and vascular health-promoting effects.[26-29]

Intrigued by these findings, researchers began exploring the anti-diabetic properties of various seaweeds, including *bladderwrack* and *Ascophyllum nodosum,* also known as *brown algae.* They discovered that these seaweeds were capable of strongly inhibiting the carbohydrate-digesting *alpha-glucosidase* enzyme in mice intestines.[28] Given to diabetic mice in the laboratory, the extracts reduced fasting glucose levels significantly at 14 days and blunted the sharp rise in blood glucose (postprandial effect) following an oral glucose tolerance test. The animals also experienced decreases in total cholesterol and sugar-damaged (glycated) protein levels.

A proprietary combination of extracts from bladderwrack and brown seaweed known as **InSea²™** has been shown to help modulate dangerous postprandial sugar swings (i.e., abrupt swings in blood sugar after eating).[25,28] Rapid swings in blood sugar after eating can increase the risk of damage to tissue proteins in the body (glycation), abdominal obesity, and food cravings that often come after a meal rich in carbohydrates.[30-32] By helping to control our postprandial blood sugar level, we can improve several aspects of metabolic health linked to body weight.

The formulator of **InSea²™** first conducted a series of studies to demonstrate the effect of the extracts on inhibiting the digestive enzymes, *amylase* and *glucosidase.* Both enzymes were powerfully inhibited within a few minutes of being exposed to the seaweed extracts. Additionally, they found that when **InSea²™** was fed to laboratory animals, glucose levels were reduced by up to **90%** following a meal compared with non-supplemented animals. Insulin levels (a measure of insulin sensitivity) were as much as **40%** lower in the **InSea²™**-supplemented mice.[33] Clearly, this supplement may provide important benefits in reducing metabolic parameters that impact both systemic health issues as well as weight gain.

Scientists found another interesting effect in the group supplemented with **InSea²™**. The normal response to an after-meal spike in blood glucose is a *surge* in **insulin** secretion. This insulin surge often causes blood glucose to be driven down too <u>low</u>. This can then create artificial hunger for more calories to elevate the depressed glucose blood levels. In lab animals taking **InSea²™**, the dramatic post-meal drop in glucose levels did <u>not</u> occur, and their glucose levels returned to baseline levels in a more gradual and natural fashion.

The after-meal drop in blood sugar produces a feeling of fatigue and can foster a sense of increased hunger leading to additional caloric intake. By "smoothing out" the postprandial sugar drop, InSea2™ exerts both biochemical and behavioral benefits on overall calorie intake. In the researchers' words, *"InSea²™ was able to change the absorption profile of a high-glycemic index (GI) food towards that of a low-GI food."*[33]

Combating the Scourge of Sucrose

Starting in early childhood, most Americans are exposed to far too much *refined* carbohydrates in the form of sucrose (table sugar). It is virtually omnipresent in processed foods. It also happens to be an enemy to human health and an age-accelerator.

Many individuals do not even knowingly ingest it. According to a 2009 study in the *Journal of Nutrition*, only **3%** of dietary sucrose is deliberately *added* by consumers; **82%** is added by manufacturers.[3] And while the World Health Organization (WHO) recommends that sucrose comprise only **10%** of total energy intake, many people substantially exceed this level from the earliest years of life—usually at the expense of key nutrients.[3,4]

Manufacturers know that most people will consistently choose sweetened over unsweetened foods and beverages.[5] People will often *continue* to do so at the expense of their own health. After years of chronic exposure to sucrose, physiological processes not unlike addiction take hold. Rapid absorption of sugars from a high-sucrose meal triggers a dangerous sequence of unfavorable hormonal and metabolic alterations that promote still greater consumption, especially in overweight individuals.[6,7] The result is the dangerously high incidence of metabolic disease we see today—obesity, type 2 diabetes, and metabolic syndrome.[8-10]

This alarming trend has led to a set of novel, evidence-based solutions. Aging individuals now have practical means at their disposal to slow or reverse the long-term consequences of chronic sucrose *overexposure.*

Sucrose is composed of two simple sugar molecules, glucose and fructose. It is poorly absorbed in the intestine in this form. In order to be utilized, it must first be broken down by the digestive enzyme **sucrase.** Blocking the enzymatic action of sucrase therefore limits uptake of *sucrose.*

Researchers have identified a potent sucrase inhibitor called **L-arabinose.** Although it is a simple plant sugar, *L-arabinose* is indigestible and <u>cannot</u> be absorbed into the blood. Instead it remains in the digestive tract and is eventually excreted.[11,12] By blocking metabolism of sucrose, *L-arabinose* inhibits the spike in blood sugar and fat synthesis that would otherwise follow a sugar-rich meal.[12] In animal models, *L-arabinose* virtually eliminates the rise in blood sugar following administration of sucrose, with blood glucose levels rising only 2% higher than in control animals that did not receive sucrose. *L-arabinose* did not exert any effect on serum glucose levels in control animals that did not receive sucrose.[13]

L-arabinose has been proven safe in both short- and long-term studies, and may contribute to lowered levels of glycosylated hemoglobin (hemoglobin A1C),[14] a measure of chronic exposure to sugar in the blood. A study combining *L-arabinose* and **white bean extract (Phaseolus vulgaris)** not only smoothed out postprandial glucose spikes and reduced insulin levels—it lowered systolic blood pressure.[14]

The Multiple Biological Effects of *Irvingia Gabonensis*

Irvingia gabonensis has been used in food preparation for millennia in Africa, where it is prized for its nutritional potential.[34,35] Based on *Irvingia's* known therapeutic properties, scientists began to examine **Irvingia** extracts for their ability to achieve glucose control.[36] The researchers found that **Irvingia** supplements produced a reduction in plasma lipid levels, especially the dangerous very low-density lipoprotein (VLDL), LDL, and triglycerides.[37] The team went on to study *Irvingia's* effect in mice, seeking to understand the molecular reasons for these impressive results.[38] What they found was that **Irvingia** produced a marked reduction in levels of a host of *amylase* enzymes, culminating in reduced absorption of glucose and concomitantly lower levels in blood and urine.

Irvingia's Mechanisms of Action

Irvingia gabonensis extract can help support weight management through multiple mechanisms of action related to carbohydrate metabolism.

These mechanisms include:

* Inhibition of *glycerol-3-phosphase dehydrogenase*, a key enzyme that helps convert sugar (glucose) to stored fat (triglyceride);

* Modulation of expression of *PPAR-gamma*, a key target that is involved in the differentiation of adipocytes (i.e. the growth and maturation of new fat cells);

* Enhancement of *adiponectin*, a protein hormone that improves insulin sensitivity and supports endothelial function;

* Inhibition of *alpha-amylase*, an enzyme that breaks down complex carbohydrate in the form of starch to maltose and dextrin;

* Modulation of *leptin*, a key hormone involved in appetite and metabolism.

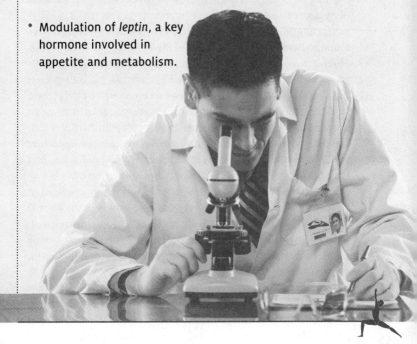

While *Irvingia* research continued to focus on its antioxidant and antimicrobial effects,[39-42] scientists began exploring its potential for combating obesity. The results of these investigations on weight loss and lipid control were eventually published.[43] In the first study, 28 people received the *Irvingia* supplement and 12 were given a placebo. All subjects stayed with their regular diets. After the month-long study period, the **Irvingia** group had lost **5.26%** of their body weight, whereas placebo recipients shed only **1.32%**. As in the older studies, supplemented patients, but not placebo patients, experienced decreases in total cholesterol, LDL, and triglycerides and an increase in HDL.

Stimulated by these findings of **Irvingia** in human trials, researchers set out to discover exactly how these effects were being obtained. They did this armed with new knowledge about the complex interactions of fat tissue in the metabolic processes, including its influence by, and on, various biochemicals involved in inflammation.[44] The researchers focused on three key elements: 1) a substance called *PPAR gamma,* produced by a gene known to contribute to human obesity; 2) the hormone *leptin* (which suppresses appetite and increases triglyceride breakdown in adipocytes); and 3) *adiponectin* (which reduces fat deposition).

Using fat cells from mice, the researchers examined the effects of *Irvingia* extract on these three important players in the obesity-generating process. After just eight days of treatment, the cells were found to have significantly reduced their production of fat stores. This occurred in response to the inhibition of an enzyme *(glycerol-3-phosphate dehydrogenase)* responsible for converting glucose to stored triglycerides in adipocytes. This was accompanied by a decrease in expression of *PPAR gamma,* with a corresponding increase in the production of the insulin-sensitizing compound *adiponectin.* The researchers concluded that, *"[Irvingia] may play an important multifaceted role in the control of adipogenesis [fat production] and have further implications in* in-vivo *anti-obesity effects."*[44]

Encouraged by these findings, the researchers progressed to larger human studies. In a recently published study in the journal *Lipids in Health and Disease,*[45] human subjects supplemented with **Irvingia** enjoyed significant improvements in body weight, body fat, and waist circumference, while their plasma lipid, adiponectin, and leptin levels all improved. Interestingly, supplemented subjects also experienced decreases in levels of the inflammatory marker **C-reactive protein,** a known cardiovascular risk factor.[45] Reduction of inflammation is now gaining the attention of scientists around the world as another important component for controlling weight and metabolic disorders. The authors' conclusion is *"Irvingia gabonensis extract may prove to be a useful tool in dealing with the emerging global epidemics of obesity, hyperlipidemia, insulin resistance, and their co-morbid conditions."*[45]

Irvingia gabonensis is one of the most exciting weight loss discoveries to date. Findings from a placebo-controlled human study showed that Irvingia caused fat loss in study participants. These participants also experienced reduced total cholesterol (by 39%), LDL (by 45%), glucose (by 32%), and triglycerides (by 45%), all markers of cardiovascular disease and type 2 diabetes.[43]

In another, larger placebo-controlled human study, participants taking *Irvingia gabonensis* lost **28 pounds** in only 10 weeks, whereas the placebo group lost virtually no weight. In addition, the Irvingia group had a waist reduction of **16.2%** versus **5.0%** in the placebo group. This study also showed that Irvingia is associated with dramatically lower levels of C-reactive protein, thereby unblocking the "leptin resistance" that causes so many weight loss programs to fail.[45] A consistent observation amongst those conducting the clinical studies was that subjects taking *Irvingia* had a diminished appetite and thus ingested fewer calories.

Summary

Scientists now recognize many biochemical pathways and control mechanisms that help regulate how we absorb, distribute, and expend ingested food throughout the body. With each new discovery, we identify additional points for intervention that can tip the scales in favor of successful reductions in body fat.

Natural supplements whose mechanisms of action are clearly understood are available to help in controlling body weight. Used responsibly and in combination, these nutrients may complement one another and have the potential to yield maximum control over abdominal fat, obesity, and cardiovascular health.

The suggested doses to be taken before the two heaviest meals of the day of the nutrients described in this chapter are:

Irvingia gabonensis extract	150 mg
Phase 3™ (*L-arabinose*)	550 mg
Phase 2™	445 mg
(*Phaseolus vulgaris*/white kidney bean extact)	
InSea™ brown seaweeds/bladderwrack)	125 mg
TeaSlender™ (Green tea phytosome)	150 mg

For consumer convenience and cost savings, all of the nutrients on the previous page (in the optimal potencies) are available without a prescription in one multi-ingredient formula.

InSea™ is a trademark of innoVactiv™. Phase 2® and Phase 3™ are used under license.

If you have any questions on the scientific content of this book, please call a Life Extension Health Advisor at 1-866-820-8083.

References:
1. *Curr Atheroscler Rep.* 2002 Nov;4(6):448-53.
2. *Eur J Clin Nutr.* 2006 Jan;60(1):18-24.
3. *Drug Metab Dispos.* 2003 May;31(5):572-9.
4. *J Med Food.* 2006 Winter;9(4):451-8.
5. *Am J Physiol Regul Integr Comp Physiol.* 2007 Jan;292(1):R77-R85.
6. *Int J Obes Relat Metab Disord.* 2000 Feb;24(2):252-8.
7. *J Nutr.* 2009 Feb;139(2):264-70.
8. *Integr Nutr.* 2008;11(2):1-14.
9. *Nutrafoods.* 2008 7(4) 21-28.
10. *Biochem Mol Biol Int.* 1998 Dec;46(5):895-903.
11. *Eur J Clin Nutr.* 2002 Dec;56(12):1186-93.
12. *J Nutr Biochem.* 2000 Jan;11(1):45-51.
13. *J Nutr Biochem.* 2007 Mar;18(3):179-83.
15. *J Nutr.* 2008 Sep;138(9):1677-83.
16. *Pflugers Arch.* 2008 Nov;457(2):293-302.
17. *Phytother Res.* 2009 Aug;23(8):1088-91.
18. *Mol Nutr Food Res.* 2009 Mar;53(3):349-60.
19. *J Am Coll Nutr.* 2007 Aug;26(4):389S-95S.
20. *Phytochemistry.* 2009 Jan;70(1):11-24.
21. *Altern Med Rev.* 2004 Mar;9(1):63-9.
22. *Yao Xue Xue Bao.* 2007 Dec;42(12):1282-7.
23. *Altern Ther Health Med.* 2007 Jul;13(4):32-7.
24. *Int J Med Sci.* 2007;4:45-52.
25. *J Ethnopharmacol.* 1989 Nov;27(1-2):35-43.
26. *Eur J Cell Biol.* 1997 Dec;74(4):376-84.
27. *J Agric Food Chem.* 2002 Feb 13;50(4):840-5.
28. *Can J Physiol Pharmacol.* 2007 Nov;85(11):1116-23.
29. *Anticancer Res.* 1996 May-Jun;16(3A):1213-8.
30. *Am J Clin Nutr.* Dec 2006;84(6):1365-73.
31. *Clin Dermatol.* 2004 Jul;22(4):310-4.
32. *Arch Intern Med.* 2006 Jul 24;166(14):1466-75.
33. http://www.innovactiv.com/index php?option=com_content&task=view&id=18&Itemid=
34. Council NR. "Dika". *Lost Crops of Africa. Vol II: Vegetables:* National Academies Press; 2006:119.
35. *J Ethnopharmacol.* 1995 Feb;45(2):125-9.
36. *Enzyme.* 1986;36(3):212-5.
37. *West Afr J Med.* 1990 Apr;9(2):108-15.
38. *Ann Nutr Metab.* 1993;37(1):14-23.
39. *J Agric Food Chem.* 2005 Aug 24;53(17):6819-24.
40. *Mol Ecol.* 2000 Jul;9(7):831-41.
41. *J Agric Food Chem.* 2002 Mar 13;50(6):1478-82.
42. *Nahrung.* 2004 Apr;48(2):85-7.
43. *Lipids Health Dis.* 2005 May 25;4:12.7.
44. *Lipids Health Dis.* 2008 Nov 13;7:44.
45. *Lipids Health Dis.* 2009 Mar 2;8:7

CHAPTER 4

Enjoy Benefits of Calorie Restriction without Hunger

The most significant **anti-aging discovery** in history was made in **1935**. In that year, rats fed a **calorie-restricted** diet achieved radically extended mean and maximum life spans, along with a delayed onset of age-related diseases.[1]

Since this finding was published 75 years ago, dozens of experiments in mammals have validated that **undernutrition *without malnutrition*** induces *profound* anti-aging effects.[2-10] Not only do calorie-restricted animals live much longer, but they remain far healthier than normally fed controls.

When a group of humans consumed a similar calorie-restricted diet, their conventional blood markers of aging (excess glucose, cholesterol, triglycerides, LDL) plummeted to much lower levels.[11,12]

In the most significant finding to date, two groups of Rhesus monkeys were studied for **20 years**. The group placed on a *moderately* restricted diet reduced their incidence of age-related disease by a **factor of three!** Cancers and cardiovascular disease were **less than half** in the *moderate* calorie-restricted group compared to controls. None of the moderate calorie-restricted group developed **diabetes** or impaired glucose tolerance, despite a usually high prevalence in these monkeys. An interesting finding showed that *moderate* calorie reduction preserved brain volume in certain regions.[13] Normal aging is accompanied by brain *shrinkage* as neurons are lost.

The Life Extension Foundation® is dedicated to providing practical options to attain many of the beneficial effects of **calorie restriction.** Our objective is to help induce the favorable changes in our members' bodies that may be responsible for the remarkable age-delaying, disease-protecting and anti-obesity effects of reduced calorie intake.

After reading this book, I hope each of you will reduce some of the excess calories you ingest each day. I can almost promise that if you do it the right way, you'll never miss those surplus *age-accelerating* sugars and fats. Even if you are unable to cut a single calorie, we have shown how you can benefit anyway by reducing the lethal impact of postprandial disorders.

We All Eat Too Much

Calorie-dense toxic foods are abundant, cheap and heavily advertised. It is no wonder that so many children and adults eat far <u>more</u> than their bodies require.

Excess calorie intake causes the bloodstream to be chronically 'bloated' with glucose, insulin, cholesterol, fat, homocysteine, and other pro-inflammatory inducers. Persistent bloodstream overload predisposes us to cancer, stroke, heart attack, senility, painful inflammation, and virtually every other age-related ailment.[15-27]

Consuming <u>excess</u> calories shortens the *average* life span by facilitating the development of *age-related diseases* that preclude us from attaining healthy longevity.

Overconsumption of calories has another insidious effect. Many scientists believe that our **life span** is largely controlled by genes that <u>program</u> our bodies to function in a youthful-healthy state. When we consume excess calories, we cause some of these genes to turn against us and contribute to *accelerated* aging and death.

If we <u>reduce</u> the amount and/or effects of ingested calories, the result is a more *favorable* gene expression profile. Such a positive effect helps us live longer, healthier lives.

Controlling the impact of *ingested* calories becomes an essential component of a science-based longevity program, as excess calorie exposure reduces life span by increasing degenerative disease risk and accelerating aging.

Reduce the Number of Calories You Absorb

Foods that are eaten must first be broken down by **digestive enzymes** before they are absorbed into the bloodstream. As we discussed in previous chapters, dietary fats are broken down by **lipase** enzymes in the stomach and small intestines. Taking 120 mg of the *lipase-inhibiting* drug **orlistat** before meals reduces dietary fat absorption by **30%**.[28]

Green and **black tea polyphenols** also inhibit **lipase**, thus enabling one to eat more calories without **absorbing** all of the fats.[29,30] In fact, when theaflavins from black tea were administered to rats, there was an immediate **suppression** of post-meal (postprandial) triglyceride elevation in the blood. The scientists attributed these results to the **"inhibition of pancreatic lipase activity."**[30]

You might think that a drug like **orlistat** that <u>reduces</u> fat absorption by **30%** would induce significant *weight loss*. The harsh reality is that study subjects must reduce their dietary fat intake <u>and</u> take orlistat to lose just **20.5 pounds** in one year. These data reveal the frightening degree to which most of us overeat.[31] In other words, even when dietary **fat** absorption is reduced by 30%, we still take in too many fat calories!

Studies show that in response to consumption of **green** or **black tea polyphenols** (or orlistat), substantial reductions in blood glucose, triglycerides, cholesterol, and other vascular risk factors occur.[32-41] These same changes happen when one reduces calorie intake,[11,12] suggesting that those who continue to eat too much should take steps to block *digestive enzymes* that enable excess calories to be absorbed.

Most Western diets contain too many refined *carbohydrates* that add to the calorie burden. Ingested *carbohydrates* are broken down for *absorption* by the enzymes **sucrase, amylase,** and **glucosidase**. One may obtain some of the effects of following a "low-carb" diet by taking 50–100 mg of a drug called acarbose (glucosidase inhibitor) before each meal.[42,43]

Nutrients that may slow carbohydrate *absorption* include **white kidney bean** (*amylase* inhibitor),[44-47] **InSea**™ (containing *amylase* and *glucosidase* inhibitors from special seaweeds),[48-51] *Irvingia* (*amylase* inhibitor)[52-55] and *L-arabinose* (sucrase inhibitor).[56]

Clinical studies confirm significant reductions in glucose, insulin, and triglyceride levels in response to taking **acarbose** alone.[57-59] These effects also occur when one restricts calorie intake. Clinical studies show dramatic reductions in heart attack rate in response to acarbose.[59] This same kind of vascular disease risk reduction has been observed in experimental studies where food intake is restricted.[60-62] What this indicates is that one may obtain some of the benefits of following a calorie-restricted diet by inhibiting *lipase, amylase, glucosidase,* <u>and</u> *sucrase* enzymes.

Consuming soluble dietary fibers before meals slows the absorption of carbohydrates, thus blunting the postprandial insulin spike.[63-66] This is another method of impeding calorie absorption and helping to mimic the effects of calorie restriction.

Improve Your Gene Expression

In response to consuming fewer calories, gene expression favoring youthful vigor is improved. Overeating, on the other hand, induces pathologic gene expression favoring the onset of diseases and accelerated aging.[72,73]

Until recently, the only way of achieving a favorable gene expression profile was through **caloric restriction**. Back in the late 1990s, research funded by the **Life Extension Foundation®** enabled scientists to compare the effects of various compounds (such as resveratrol) to the *gene expression* changes that occur during calorie restriction.

These experiments have been used to identify *nutrients* that mimic many of the beneficial gene expression changes observed during **calorie restriction**. If you are a health-conscious individual, you will be pleased to know that some of the nutrients you are taking (such as fish oil and vitamin D) favorably influence *gene expression*. Other nutrients that have demonstrated profound calorie restriction mimetic effects on gene expression include pterostilbene (a blueberry extract), quercetin, and fisetin (a strawberry extract).

Once scientists gain total control over the expression of the genes that affect longevity, mankind may achieve biological immortality. Until that time arrives, it is comforting to know that we can now exert at least some control over the expression of genes that influence our health and longevity.

With the discovery of *novel plant extracts* that mimic some of the *gene expression* changes observed in response to *calorie restriction*, one may enjoy many of the longevity benefits of undereating by taking the proper supplements daily.

Moderate Calorie Restriction — It's Not as Difficult as You Think!

At the beginning of this chapter we described the Rhesus monkey study that utilized only modest calorie restriction to achieve remarkable longevity benefits. From everything we know today, it would appear that many of you could migrate towards a routine of at least modest calorie reduction and feel better doing so.

For too many people, copious food intake has become an addictive drug. Fortunately, there are safe ways to suppress appetite using **Irvingia**, **metformin,** and/or a plant extract discovered in Europe called **pinolenic acid** that has been shown to suppress appetite without causing any stimulatory effect.

Pinolenic acid is a polyunsaturated fatty acid derived from pine nuts. It attacks the underlying mechanisms involved in hunger so effectively that study participants reduced their food intake by **36%**.[85]

Pinolenic acid stimulates the secretion of the hunger-suppressing hormones *cholecystokinin* (CCK)[86] and *glucagon-like peptide-1* (GLP-1). The results from human clinical studies using pinolenic acid reveal a reduced "desire to eat" along with early satiety.[85] Those seeking to curb their appetite to reduce daily calorie intake should take **three 1000 mg** capsules of a pinolenic acid before most meals.

Practical Options to Emulate Calorie Restriction

The scientific data solidly document that surplus calorie intake shortens your life span.[87,88] Everyone responds differently when reducing food intake. But most people can at least <u>modestly</u> decrease the number of calories they consume each day.

Most individuals, however, will still eat more than they should. Fortunately, there are multiple ways to inhibit the activity of *digestive enzymes,* and thus spare most of the body from the lethal effects of excess calorie <u>absorption</u>. An aggressive, initial three-month plan to reduce the number of absorbed calories may include the following nutrients and medications:

Orlistat (Inhibits *lipase* enzyme*[28,31,35,40,41])	120 mg
Acarbose	50-100 mg
(Inhibits alpha-*glucosidase enzyme*[42,43,57,59])	
Irvingia gabonensis extract	150 mg
Phase 3™ (*L-arabinose*)	550 mg
Phase 2™	445 mg
(*Phaseolus vulgaris*/white kidney bean extract)	
InSea™ brown seaweeds/bladderwrack)	125 mg
TeaSlender™(Green tea phytosome)	150 mg
Black tea theaflavins	300–350 mg
(Theaflavins also inhibit lipase, but not as potently as orlistat.[30])	

For some individuals, drugs like **orlistat** and **acarbose** will cause gastrointestinal discomfort after eating too much. One objective of suggesting a 90-day trial using these drugs is to forcibly educate you about healthier lifelong dietary patterns. For example, if you continue to consume excess calories, you may experience digestive discomforts when taking these digestive enzyme-blocking drugs. Understanding that calories that are remaining in your digestive tract were destined to be absorbed into your bloodstream (which will increase your risk of metabolic disease and may significantly shorten your life) may motivate you to eat less.

In case you have not figured this out yet, a side benefit to doing all this is a loss of surplus body fat.

We Live in an Exciting Era!

Scientists continue to validate the health benefits of nutrients that **Life Extension** members supplement with every day. Only recently, however, have these favorable effects been linked to the ability of these nutrients to mimic *gene expression* changes that occur in response to **calorie restriction**.[72, 101-105]

An explosive volume of newly published research indicates that aging humans can exert tremendous degrees of *control* as to whether they maintain *youthful* or *senescent* gene expression patterns in their cellular DNA.[106-108]

Some youthful gene expression can be maintained by reducing intake of calories to a level **20–40%** lower than is typical, while still obtaining all the necessary nutrients and vitamins.[13,109-113] The most recent Rhesus monkey study indicates even a *modest* calorie-restricted diet produces **huge reductions** in degenerative disease.[13]

Those who are unable to sufficiently cut their food intake can still inhibit the *absorption* of ingested calories by taking compounds (such as **orlistat, acarbose,** and/or nutrients that funciton via similar mechanisms) that block *digestive enzyme* activity.

Finally, and most exciting of all, there are nutrients (such as **pterostilbene** and **resveratrol**) that have been shown to mimic many of the favorable effects induced by **calorie restriction**.[102-104,114-116] These low-cost nutrients provide humans with an unprecedented power to determine whether their cellular DNA expresses **youth-promoting** or **senescent-inducing** genes. Humans have never enjoyed so much control over the rate that they age!

This book has two missions. One is to enable those who seriously want to lose weight to achieve a healthy result. The other is to provide a substantial risk reduction in virtually every age-related disease, as so many of them are directly related to one's body weight.

As your body is purged of excess fat pounds, you should be comforted in knowing your odds of contracting most cancers, heart attack, stroke, arthritis, type 2 diabetes, and liver failure has been drastically lowered.

If you have any questions on the scientific content of this book, please call a Life Extension Health Advisor at 1-866-820-8083.

References:

1. *Nutrition*. 1989 May-Jun;5(3):155-71.
2. *Science*. 1982 Mar 12;215(4538):1415-8.
3. *J Nutr*. 1986 Apr;116(4):641-54.
4. *J Nutr Health Aging*. 1999;3(2):102-10.
5. *Eur J Clin Nutr*. 2000 Jun;54 Suppl 3:S15-20.
6. *J Nutr Health Aging*. 1999; 3(2):69-76.
7. *Physiol Behav*. 1997 Jul;62(1):97-103.
8. *Am J Physiol Endocrinol Metab*. 2005 May;288(5):E965-72.
9. *Exp Gerontol*. 1992 Sep-Dec;27(5-6):575-81.
10. *J Gerontol*. 1989 Nov;44(6):67-71.
11. *Physiol Behav*. 2009 Mar 23;96(4-5):703-8.
12. *Atherosclerosis*. 2009 Mar;203(1):206-13.
13. *Science*. 2009 Jul 10;325(5937):201-4.
14. *J Clin Psych*. 2002;58(4).
15. *Asia Pac J Clin Nutr*. 2007;16(4):671-6.
16. *Curr Hypertens Rep*. 2008 Feb;10(1):32-8.
17. *JAMA*. 2002 Dec 4;288(21):2709-16.
18. *Prev Med*. 2006 May;42(5):336-42.
19. *Cell*. 2008 Oct 3;135(1):61-73.
20. *Med Sci* (Paris). 2005 Dec;21 Spec No10-8.
21. *Mol Med*. 2009 Jul-Aug;15(7-8):228-34.
22. *Am J Physiol Heart Circ Physiol*. 2007 Feb;292(2):H904-11.
23. *Curr Med Res Opin*. 2005 Jul;21(7):989-98.
24. *Curr Drug Targets Inflamm Allergy*. 2004 Dec;3(4):455-8.
25. *Lancet*. 2005 Apr 16-22;365(9468):1415-28.
26. *J Nutr Biochem*. 2008 Aug;19(8):491-504.
27. *BMJ*. 2007 Dec 1;335(7630):1134.
28. *Drugs*. 2006 66(12):1625-56.
29. *J Nutr Biochem*. 2000 Jan;11(1):45-51.
30. *J Agric Food Chem*. 2009;57(15):7131-6.
31. *Eat Weight Disord*. 2006 Mar;11(1):e35-41.
32. *Diabetes Care*. 2003 26:1714-8.
33. *Eur J Clin Nutr*. 2008 Aug;62(8):953-60.
34. *J Lipid Res*. 2007 Nov;48(11):2334-43.
35. *Atherosclerosis*. 2007 Aug;193(2):428-37.
36. *J Hypertens*. 1999 Apr;17(4):457-63.
37. *QJM*. 2001 May;94(5):277-82.
38. *Obesity* (Silver Spring). 2007 Jun;15(6):1473-83.
39. *Inflammopharmacology*. 2008 Oct;16(5):230-4.
40. *Obes Res*. 2000 Jan;8(1):49-61.
41. *Diabet Med*. 2005 Dec;22(12):1737-43.
42. *J Atheroscler Thromb*. 2008 Jun;15(3):154-9.
43. *Stroke*. 2004 May;35(5):1073-8.
44. *Altern Ther Health Med*. 2007 Jul-Aug;13(4):32-7.
45. *Int J Med Sci*. 2007 Jan 24;4(1):45-52.
46. *Yao Xue Xue Bao*. 2007 Dec;42(12):1282-7.
47. *Altern Med Rev*. 2004 Mar;9(1):63-9.
48. *J Ethnopharmacol*. 1989 Nov;27(1-2):35-43.
49. *Plant Foods Hum Nutr*. 2008 Dec;63(4):163-9.
50. *Can J Physiol Pharmacol*. 2007 Nov;85(11):1116-23.
51. Available at: http://www.naturalproductsinsider.com/news/2009/12/insea2-reduces-glycemic-response.aspx#. Accessed December 2, 2009.
52. *Ann Nutr Metab*. 1993; 37(1):14-23.
53. *Lipids Health Dis*. 2008 Mar 31;7:12.
54. *Lipids Health Dis*. 2009 Mar 2;8:7.
55. *Lipids Health Dis*. 2008 Nov 13;7:44.
56. *J Nutr*. 2001:131:796-9.
57. *Int J Cardiol*. 2006 Feb 8;107(1):11-20.
58. Aronson JK. Meyler's Side Effects of Endocrine and Metabolic Drugs. New York, NY: Elsevier Science; 2009.
59. *Eur Heart J*. 2004 Jan;25(1):10-6.
60. *Circ Res*. 2008 Mar 14;102(5):519-28.

61. *Am J Physiol Endocrinol Metab.* 2007 Jul;293(1):E197-202.
62. *Proc Natl Acad Sci U S A.* 2004 Apr 27;101(17):6659-63.
63. *Med Hypotheses.* 2002 Jun;58(6):487-90.
64. *Am J Clin Nutr.* 2003 Nov;78(5):920-7.
65. *Am J Ther.* 2007 Mar;14(2):203-12.
66. *Asia Pac J Clin Nutr.* 2007;16(1):16-24.
67. *J Indian Med Assoc.* 2005 Nov;103(11):594-5.
68. *Am J Med.* 2006 May;119(5 Suppl 1):S10-6.
69. *Exp Clin Endocrinol Diabetes.* 2005 Feb;113(2):80-4.
70. *N Engl J Med.* 1996 Jan 25;334(4):269-70.
71. *Eur J Clin Invest.* 1998 Jun;28(6):441-6.
72. *Nutr Rev.* 2007 Dec;65(12 Pt 2):S203-7.
73. *J Nutr Health Aging.* 1999 3(2):102-10.
74. *Curr Drug Targets Inflamm Allergy.* 2004 Dec;3(4):455-8.
75. *Cancer Epidemiol Biomarkers Prev.* 2006 Feb;15(2):334-41.
76. *Rinsho Byori.* 1999 Jun;47(6):554-60.
77. *Int J Cancer.* 1996 Dec 11;68(6):716-22.
78. *Cancer Epidemiol Biomarkers Prev.* 2006 Dec;15(12):2453-60.
79. *J Gerontol A Biol Sci Med Sci.* 2009 Apr 6.
80. *JAMA.* 2006 Apr 5;295(13):1539-48.
81. *JAMA.* 2002 Dec 4;288(21):2709-16.
82. *Circulation.* 2005 Aug 2;112(5):666-73.
83. *Nat Rev Cancer.* 2004 Aug;4(8):579-91.
84. *Neural Plast.* 2005;12(4):311-28.
85. *Lipids Health Dis.* 2008 Mar 20;7:10.
86. *Obes Rev.* 2005 Nov;6(4):297-306.
87. *JAMA.* 2005 Apr 20;293(15):1861-7.
88. *JAMA.* 2003 Jan 8;289(2):187-93.
89. *Am J Clin Nutr.* 2009 Aug;90(2):415-24.
90. *J Steroid Biochem Mol Biol.* 2007 Mar;103(3-5):538-45.
91. *Cell.* 2006 Dec 15;127(6):1109-22.
92. *Cancer Res.* 2008 Sep 15;68(18):7428-38.
93. *Anticancer Res.* 2009 Sep;29(9):3585-90.
94. *Crit Care Med.* 2004 Oct;32(10):2097-103.
95. *J Agric Food Chem.* 1999 Apr;47(4):1416-21.
96. *Eur J Pharmacol.* 1999 Feb 19;367(2-3):379-88.
97. *Arch Pharm Res.* 2002 Oct;25(5):561-71.
98. *Lancet Oncol.* 2000 Nov;1:181-8.
99. *Nutr Cancer.* 1999;35(1):80-6.
100. *Anticancer Agents Med Chem.* 2006 Sep;6(5):389-406.
101. *Free Radic Biol Med.* 2004 Apr 15;36(8):1043-57.
102. *Cell Metab.* 2008 Aug;8(2):157-68.
103. *Nature.* 2006 Nov 16;444(7117):337-42.
104. *PLoS One.* 2008 Jun 4;3(6):e2264.
105. *OMICS.* 2008 Dec;12(4):251-61.
106. *Minerva Pediatr.* 2008 Aug;60(4):443-55.
107. *Curr Opin Lipidol.* 2008 Jun;19(3):242-7.
108. *Nutrition.* 2007 Nov;23(11-12):844-52.
109. *Cell Mol Life Sci.* 2007 Jun;64(11):1323-8.
110. *Cell.* 2005 Feb 25;120(4):473-82.
111. *Cell Mol Life Sci.* 2007;64:752-67.
112. *Trends Mol Med.* 2007;13:64-71.
113. *Exp Gerontol.* 2009;44:70-4.
114. *J Agric Food Chem.* 2002 Jun 5;50(12):3453-7.
115. *J Agric Food Chem.* 2008 Nov 26;56(22):10544-51.
116. *Mol Nutr Food Res.* 2008 Jun;52 Suppl 1:S62-70.

CHAPTER 5

Improve Your Sleep and Take Off Weight

In case you weren't aware, sleep deprivation increases both your appetite and your risk of diabetes ... two things you definitely want under control in any weight loss program. Good, refreshing sleep is essential for your health and well-being.

Yet imsomnia is rampant in the industrialized world. A recently published survey indicates that it afflicts slightly more than 27 percent of adults in the United States.[3] Studies show that poor sleepers receive fewer promotions, have increased rates of absenteeism, and tend to demonstrate poor productivity.[1,2]

In an international study of insomniacs, the most common complaint was poor "sleep maintenance," cited by 73 percent, while difficulty falling asleep came in second, at 61 percent. About half the study participants (48 percent) cited "poor sleep quality" as their predominant symptom.[3]

Not surprisingly, a majority of insomniacs studied are "somewhat" or "very" bothered by their insomnia, noting that it adversely impacted their daily quality of life.[3] Insomnia often results in daytime sleepiness, reduced cognitive performance, and potentially dangerous inattentiveness.

One recent study, conducted in Brazil, found that an alarming 22 percent of long-haul truckers had fallen asleep at the wheel, with nearly 3% falling asleep on the job daily.[4]

There is no single patient type when it comes to poor sleep, although women tend to suffer from insomnia in greater numbers than men.

Insomnia may be associated with a wide variety of prescription drugs and other conditions, such as Parkinson's disease, Alzheimer's disease, coronary artery disease, cancer, dementia, breathing difficulties (e.g., sleep apnea), or chronic conditions such as rheumatism.[5,6]

To better understand the connection between insomnia and diseases, researchers have conducted studies examining the levels of various chemical signals (called cytokines) in sleep and insomnia. They have discovered that nighttime secretion of the cytokine interleukin-6 is significantly increased in patients with primary insomnia.[7] Interleukin-6 is a pro-inflammatory cytokine linked to cardiovascular and other diseases. Researchers have found that lack of sleep correlates with interleukin-6 production both day and night, which might explain why so many insomniacs experience daytime sleepiness. Interleukin-6 is involved in regulating sleep.[8]

Additional studies have found that tumor necrosis factor, another pro-inflammatory cytokine, is increased in insomniacs during the daytime and that levels of these two cytokines are closely related to the level of fatigue experienced.[9] These findings mean that insomnia may promote a constant state of low-grade inflammation that may accelerate many diseases of aging, including obesity.

Sleep and Aging

As people age, their sleep gradually becomes more disjointed, shallower, and shorter. Sleep cycles through phases throughout the night. Early stage-1 sleep is the lightest stage. Delta sleep, or stage-4 sleep, is the deepest and most refreshing phase. During stage-1 sleep, we are easily awakened; during delta sleep, the reverse is true. Unfortunately, delta sleep declines in the elderly.[10] This age-related change in delta sleep may explain why sleep tends to be fragmentary in the elderly. Interestingly, there is little change throughout life in the amount of REM (rapid eye movement) sleep. REM sleep is the active phase of sleep where the brain is still very active. Although they get less sleep and may waken exceptionally early, the elderly often suffer from daytime drowsiness because of this altered sleep architecture. Many think that older individuals simply require less sleep than others, however, there is no evidence to support this belief. The fact that older adults sleep less than younger adults may actually reflect their inability, rather than their need, to sleep.[2]

Melatonin and Sleep

Melatonin is a hormone released by the pineal gland in response to the absence of light. Its release into the bloodstream triggers a chain of events that promotes sleep. It is well-known for this role and may be used effectively as an oral supplement to help re-entrain the sleep cycle in situations such as jet lag, in which the normal circadian rhythm of sleeping and waking gets out of sync with the local environment.[11,12,13] Melatonin production decreases during aging, and patients with Alzheimer's disease exhibit a profound decrease in this important hormone. When Alzheimer's patients are given melatonin orally, their sleep improves and the progression of cognitive impairment slows.[14] The natural decline in melatonin may be the underlying cause of disturbances in sleep architecture among the elderly.[15,16] Studies of its mechanism of action suggest that melatonin triggers a drop in body temperature through a complex interaction with the hypothalamic-pituitary-thyroid axis and by stimulation or suppression of certain corollary hormones, which in turn is associated with the onset of sleep. Melatonin is also believed to potentiate the effects of the neurotransmitter most associated with sleep and relaxation, gamma-aminobutyric acid (GABA), through direct interaction with GABA receptors.[17,18,19] More recent data indicate that melatonin may, in fact, be directly sleep-inducing.[20] In light of the research demonstrating melatonin's many roles in the body, it seems that a deficiency of this hormone could pose health risks. For instance, there appears to be a relationship between the age-related decline in melatonin production and the decline in immune function that also accompanies old age. Known as immunosenescence, this phenomenon is associated with an increased incidence of cancer and infectious disease. As a result, some scientists have proposed that melatonin may be useful to enhance immunity and reduce the incidence and severity of these age-related maladies.[21] One researcher stated, "Chronic sleep loss could contribute to acceleration of the aging process."[22]

Despite these positive reports, many people require more than just melatonin to achieve optimal sleep.

Sleep Hygiene

Virtually everyone will struggle with insomnia on occasion. For instance, a 1995 poll of Americans found that 49 percent were dissatisfied with their sleep at least five nights each month.[23] The first step to ensuring adequate sleep is to implement good sleep hygiene. Sleep hygiene refers to a set of behaviors designed to encourage routine, restful sleep. These behaviors include some obvious elements, such as choosing a dark, quiet sleeping environment, avoiding caffeine or other stimulants (including nicotine) in the hours preceding bedtime, and keeping an unchanging bedtime-wake schedule. It is especially important to set a schedule and stick to it. Doctors recommend going to bed and rising at the same times every day, even on weekends. They also recommend reserving the bedroom for sleep; do not bring work to bed or watch

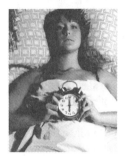

television, for example. Regular exercise is known to improve sleep,[24] but it should not be done immediately before retiring, when it may have a stimulating rather than a sedating effect. Experts also recommend finding ways to manage stress and reduce worries so that bedtime is a more relaxing experience.[25] Do not nap during the day if doing so seems to make it harder to fall asleep at night, and consider eating a tryptophan-rich snack before bedtime (e.g., whole-grain cereal with milk, yogurt with fresh fruit). Avoid foods, such as chocolate, that may contain caffeine. Limit intake of alcohol. Although it may hasten sleep, evidence suggests that it interferes with deep, restful sleep.[25,26, 27] In fact, in one study of middle-aged men, a "moderate" dose of alcohol (defined as 0.55 g ethanol per kilogram of body weight) taken six hours before scheduled bedtime was enough to significantly alter the restfulness of sleep. Despite having zero breath-alcohol concentrations at bedtime, the men's sleep efficiency, total sleep time, stage 1, and REM sleep were all reduced. In the second half of the sleep episode, wakefulness increased twofold. Although they had metabolized and effectively eliminated the alcohol they had consumed in late afternoon, the men clearly suffered significant disruptions in subsequent sleep quality.[28]

Transient Insomnia/Chronic Insomnia

For some individuals, problems falling or remaining asleep become chronic. Defined as "inadequate quantity or quality of sleep that has persisted for at least one month,"[2] chronic insomnia is often characterized by an individual's primary complaint: Does the patient experience more difficulty falling asleep or staying asleep? Effective treatment of insomnia relies on understanding the causes of particular symptoms.

It should be noted that certain medical conditions, such as menopause, depression, allergies, arthritis, or benign prostatic hypertrophy, may affect sleep quality. Common medications may add to the problem. It may be prudent to address such underlying conditions before, or in addition to, addressing insomnia. Menopausal women, for example, may benefit from treatment with supplements, such as maca root (*Lepidium peruvianum*) which has been shown to provide significant support to women undergoing menopause, i.e., reduced hot flashes, night sweats, and better mood, thus improving sleep.[29-31]

Difficulty Staying Asleep

One subtype of chronic insomnia is typified by the inability to remain asleep throughout the night despite falling asleep with little or no difficulty. Chronic drug or alcohol abuse is one cause; depression and anxiety disorders are other potential causes. Breathing disorders are also linked with chronic insomnia. Upper airway resistance syndrome may interfere with restful sleep, and obstructive sleep apnea syndrome, which frequently occurs in obese patients, may be characterized by loud snoring, choking, or gasping episodes during sleep. These frequent nocturnal breathing interruptions fragment sleep. As a result, both conditions are accompanied by excessive daytime drowsiness. Breathing disorders may require diagnosis in a sleep laboratory and may warrant special treatment. For instance, continuous positive airway pressure treatment (using a type of breathing mask) may be prescribed to treat sleep apnea. Such treatments may greatly improve sleep.[32] Sleep apnea patients should avoid any medications, such as sedatives or hypnotics that may depress the respiratory system. These medications include barbiturates (e.g., Seconal® and Nembutol®) and benzodiazepines (e.g., Valium®).[2]

Natural Remedies For Insomnia

Even with adequate sleep hygiene, many people — especially elderly people — still have trouble sleeping. Many doctors are quick to prescribe any of the dozens of medications that are currently used as potential sleep aids. While some of the newer generation of "sleeping pills" may be safer and less habit forming than older medications, natural remedies are a better first-line therapy.

Valerian. Preparations made from the roots of valerian *(Valeriana officinalis)* have long been relied on to hasten refreshing sleep. Controlled studies show that valerian decreases the amount of time it takes to fall asleep, as well as the subjective quality of sleep, compared to a placebo. Valerian also improves quality of sleep; at least one study has shown that valerian increases the percentage of time participants spend in slow-wave sleep. This is significant because slow-wave sleep is considered the most profoundly refreshing sleep phase.[33,34,35,36] One recent multicenter, double-blind, randomized parallel group study compared valerian, 600 mg/day, to the commonly prescribed tranquilizer oxazepam (Serax®). Valerian was at least as effective.[38]

While valerian is generally considered safe,[39] the same cannot be said of most hypnotic drugs. "Long-term use of hypnotic agents can become complicated by drug tolerance, dependence, or rebound insomnia," noted one scientist.[40] Prescription drugs such as Valium® may cause morning "hangover": fogginess of the mind, lethargy, clumsiness, and other symptoms. Valerian has consistently been shown to have no such side effects. In a randomized, controlled, double-blind study, researchers administered 600 mg valerian extract to 102 participants. The following morning, participants' reaction times, alertness, and concentration were evaluated. Researchers found no negative effects on any objective parameters of alertness or ability to concentrate subsequent to single or multiple doses of valerian.[41] More recently, researchers examined the effects of exceptionally high doses of valerian (up to 1800 mg) on parameters relating to "hangover" versus diazepam (Valium®) or placebo. The researchers concluded that valerian extract had no significant effects on any of the dependent measures. In contrast, the prescription drug impaired cognitive performance and affected mood.[42]

Traditionally, patients have been advised to take valerian for up to two weeks before expecting it to become fully effective. It is unclear whether this is truly necessary, however, as the clinical evidence is contradictory.[43] Valerian contains the amino acid GABA, which could directly cause sedation. GABA acts as a neurotransmitter involved in regulation of relaxation, anxiety, and sleep. Valerian is also known to interact with GABA already active in the brain. Valerian prompts the release of GABA and inhibits enzymes involved in GABA's breakdown, thus further increasing levels of this "relaxation neurotransmitter".[44,45]

Although it does not regulate sale or production of valerian, the Food and Drug Administration (FDA) lists valerian as "Generally Recognized as Safe." No significant drug interactions have been reported although valerian might increase the sedating effects of barbiturates or anesthesia drugs.[45] It is also possible, although not definitively established, that valerian affects the metabolism of some other drugs in a manner similar to grapefruit.[46,47] Valerian has also been associated with liver damage although purified extract of valerian appears to be safe for the liver. Most published studies have found valerian effective for the treatment of insomnia when root extract equivalent to 300 to 600 mg is taken 30 minutes to two hours before a person's intended bedtime. A study of valerian pharmacokinetics — the rate at which active constituents enter the bloodstream and are subsequently eliminated from the body — confirmed the effectiveness of this dosing regimen.[48]

(Continued on page 86)

Good Sleep Hygiene

Getting a good night's sleep starts with good sleep hygiene. Experts recommend the following:

- Go to bed and rise at the same times every day, even on weekends.
- Maintain a bedtime routine, doing the same (relaxing) activities every night.
- Do not use the bed for anything but sleep and sex.
- Sleep in a dark, quiet room. If necessary, mask ambient noises with a fan or other "white-noise" generator. Or try earplugs.
- If you have not fallen asleep after 30 minutes, get up and sit quietly in another room. Do not fret about your lack of sleep. After 20 minutes, retire to bed again. Repeat as necessary. Known as stimulus control therapy, this approach to falling asleep helps reassociate the bedroom with restful sleep rather than stress over lack of sleep.
- Avoid caffeine, tobacco, and alcohol in the hours preceding bedtime.
- Exercise routinely during the day to improve onset and quality of sleep.
- Avoid napping during the day.

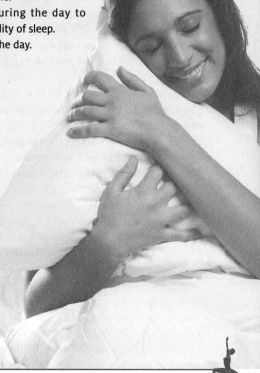

L-tryptophan. L-tryptophan is an amino acid that serves as a precursor for the neurotransmitter serotonin. Serotonin has been implicated in the regulation of sleep, depression, anxiety, appetite, sexual behavior, and body temperature.[49] In recent years, researchers have studied L-tryptophan's ability to help insomniacs. One study found that tryptophan depletion contributed to insomnia. The researchers gave 15 insomniacs an amino acid drink that depleted tryptophan, then studied the participants' sleep patterns. They found that sleep was significantly disrupted after tryptophan levels were lowered.[50] Another study comparing "protein-source" tryptophan, or tryptophan that comes from a protein, with pharmaceutical-grade tryptophan, which does not include protein, found they were equally effective in treating insomnia.[51] Previously, it was thought that protein-source tryptophan would be less effective because protein contains amino acids that interfere with tryptophan's transport into the brain.

Lemon balm. Lemon balm *(Melissa officinalis L)* is often paired with valerian. A recently published study of a combination of valerian and lemon balm for the treatment of restlessness and disordered sleep in children found "a distinct and convincing reduction in severity ... for all symptoms in the investigators' and parents' ratings."[52] About 81 percent of patients with sleep disorders experienced improvement of their symptoms after taking the study preparation.

Lemon balm appears to work by reducing anxiety. A recent double-blind, placebo-controlled, randomized, balanced crossover experiment showed that a 600-mg dose of lemon balm improved the negative mood effects of a standardized procedure designed to induce stress under laboratory conditions. Participants taking lemon balm had "significantly increased self-ratings of calmness," noted the researchers. "In addition, a significant increase in the speed of mathematical processing, with no reduction in accuracy, was observed after ingestion of the 300-mg dose."[53]

Prescription Sleep Aids

Ideally, prescription drugs are not necessary for sleep aid. Some of these medications carry a risk of tolerance. In other words, it requires more and more of the medication to get a good night's rest. Another side effect is daytime drowsiness caused by lingering effects from the previous night's medication. Worse yet, many of these medications are addictive in the sense that patients lose the ability to sleep without them. However, if natural remedies fail to bring about refreshing sleep, it is Life Extension's position that people should use whatever means are available to them, including prescription medications, to get good sleep. Sleep medications may be classified into the following categories:

Benzodiazepines. These drugs were introduced in the 1960s and were used for the treatment of insomnia. They were very popular sleep aids for several decades but are prescribed less frequently today because of concerns over dependency, impairment in memory and movement, and a "hangover" effect the next day. The following are some popular benzodiazepines:

- Valium® (diazepam)
- Dalmane® (flurazepam)
- Doral® (quazepam)
- Halcion® (triazolam)
- ProSom® (estazolam)
- Restoril® (temazepam)
- Klonopin® (clonazepam)

Nonbenzodiazepine, benzodiazepine receptor agonists. Introduced in the 1990s and sometimes referred to as "Z drugs," these drugs are now the first-line treatment for insomnia. They include Ambien® (zolpidem) and Sonata® (zaleplon). These drugs have been shown to reduce the time it takes to fall asleep and have fewer side effects than the benzodiazepines, but they are also recommended for short-term use. In general, however, most researchers call for better long-term studies. Other drugs used to treat insomnia include sedative antidepressants, such as trazodone (Desyrel®), amitriptyline (Elavil®) and doxepin (Sinequan®). These medications are usually prescribed for insomnia in the context of depression rather than for treatment of primary insomnia, at least in part because of their many side effects, including dry mouth, weight gain, constipation, and a host of other problems. A typical dose of Elavil® taken a few hours before bedtime is 10 to 25 mg. Some people use Elavil® until the side effects become too pronounced and then discontinue it for months or years. The problem with drugs like Elavil® (amitriptyline) is that they increase hunger and can induce profound weight gain. Those seeking to lose weight should avoid any kind of tricyclic antidepressant drug.

One way of avoiding the tolerance problem is to alternate the type of sleeping pill used. Here is a suggested prescription drug schedule to treat chronic insomnia for the person who has never taken prescription sleeping pills:

1. Valium, 2.5 mg, taken only at bedtime for 30 days
2. During the next 30-day cycle, 5 to 10 mg Ambien® taken only at bedtime
3. During the next 30-day cycle, 1 to 3 mg Klonopin® taken only at bedtime

At some point, patients may find that they do better by taking Valium® one night, Ambien® the next night, and Klonopin® the third night. The drug Sonata® in a 5 to 10 mg dose provides about 5 hours of sleep and can be helpful on occasions when only a limited amount of sleep time is available. If heavy alcohol is consumed, these types of drugs should be avoided on the same night. It should be noted that chronic alcohol intake in and of itself is a major cause of poor sleep patterns. A person with chronic insomnia must develop a close relationship with a physician who understands that some people need sleep medications on a routine basis or their lives will be miserable and that they are also at a higher risk of contracting a serious degenerative disease. Melatonin may help any of these prescription drugs work more effectively.

Life Extension Foundation Recommendations

Chronic insomnia is best approached by behavior modification and natural therapies before turning to prescription drugs. The following lifestyle changes may relieve insomnia:

- Avoid caffeine at least six hours before bedtime.
- Avoid smoking for six hours before bedtime.
- Get regular exercise, but do not exercise within three hours of bedtime.
- Establish regular bedtime and waking hours.
- Do not work in the bedroom.
- Consider using white-noise generators or relaxing music to "turn off" your mind.
- Sleep in a completely dark room.
- Avoid alcohol most days and nights.

If sleep is disrupted by another condition, such as restless legs syndrome, painful arthritis, or carpal tunnel syndrome, it may be helpful to seek treatment for that condition. In addition, the following herbs and supplements have been shown to help induce sleep:

- **Valerian**—300 to 600 milligrams (mg) valerian root 30 minutes to two hours before bedtime. If taking liquid valerian, take 30 to 40 drops of extract in a small amount of warm water within the hour before bedtime. Long-term valerian therapy is not recommended. Valerian is sometimes used with lemon balm.
- **Melatonin**—300 micrograms (mcg) to 10 mg about 30 minutes before bedtime. Sometimes lower doses work better than higher doses.
- **GABA**—350 to 700 mg before bedtime (taken sublingually).
- **L-tryptophan**—1500 to 2000 mg before bedtime in combination with nutrients that protect absorbed tryptophan from degradation in the bloodstream before it can cross the blood-brain barrier to produce calming serotonin. Refer to www.lef.org/tryptophan for details.

If natural sleep remedies do not restore refreshing sleep, pharmaceutical drugs are available, including Klonopin®, Ambien®, Lunesta®, and many others. These drugs must be prescribed by a physician. In addition, dehydroepiandrosterone (DHEA) replacement therapy may be recommended. Almost all aging humans are deficient in DHEA, and DHEA may help reduce cortisol levels and produce a feeling of well-being. Although DHEA has not been studied in insomnia, a suggested starting dose of 15 to 75 mg, followed by blood testing after three to six weeks, is recommended to promote peace of mind. It is important to take DHEA in the morning as taking it at night can be stimulatory.

Insomnia Safety Caveats

An aggressive program of dietary supplementation should not be launched without the supervision of a qualified physician. Several of the nutrients suggested in this protocol may have adverse effects. These include:

L-Tryptophan
- Do not take L-tryptophan if you have carcinoid tumors.
- Do not take L-tryptophan while taking monoamine oxidase inhibitors (MAOIs) (type A) or within 2 weeks of discontinuing MAOIs.

- Do not take L-tryptophan with any antidepressant medications, including selective serotonin reuptake inhibitors (SSRIs), tricyclic antidepressants or MAOIs.
- Do not take L-tryptophan with serotonin 5-HT receptor agonists, including naratriptan, sumatriptan and zolmitriptan.
- Do not take L-tryptophan if you have ischemic heart disease (e.g., a history of myocardial infarction, angina pectoris or documented silent ischemia), coronary artery spasm (e.g., Prinzmetal sangina), uncontrolled hypertension or any other significant cardiovascular disease.

Melatonin

- Do not take melatonin if you are depressed.
- Do not take high doses of melatonin if you are trying to conceive. High doses of melatonin have been shown to inhibit ovulation.
- Melatonin can cause morning grogginess, a feeling of having a hangover or a "heavy head," or gastrointestinal symptoms such as nausea and diarrhea.

If you have any questions on the scientific content of this book, please call a Life Extension Health Advisor at 1-866-820-8083.

References
1. *Soc Sci Med.* 1991;33:127–37.
2. *Am Fam Physician.* 1999 Oct 1;60(5):1431–8; discussion 1441–2.
3. *Curr Med Res Opin.* 2005 Nov;21(11):1785–92.
4. *Public Health.* 2005 Oct;119(10):925–9.
5. *J Support Oncol.* 2005 Sep-Oct;3(5):349–59.
6. *Arthritis Rheum.* 2005 Dec 15;53(6):911–9.
7. *Brain Behav Immun.* 2005 Aug 3.
8. *Neuroimmunomodulation.* 2005;12(3):131–40. Review.
9. *Metabolism.* 2002 Jul;51(7):887–92.
10. *N Engl J Med.* 1974;290:487–99.
11. *J Biol Rhythms.* 2003 Aug;18(4):318–28.
12. *Sleep.* 2005 Jan 1;28(1):33–44.
13. *Med Hypotheses.* 2004;63(6):1074–80.
14. *Acta Pharmacol Sin.* 2006 Jan;27(1):41–9.
15. *Neurobiol Aging.* 2005 Oct;26(9):1307–19.
16. *Exp Gerontol.* 2005 Dec;40(12):911–25.
17. *J Pineal Res.* 2005 Nov;39(4):353–9.
18. *Neuro Endocrinol Lett.* 2004 Oct;25(5):368–72.
19. *Altern Med Rev.* 2005 Dec;10(4):326–36.
20. *J Clin Psychiatry.* 2005 Mar;66(3):384–90.
21. *Immun Ageing.* 2005 Nov 29;2:17.

22. *Essent Psychopharmacol.* 2005;6(6):341–7.
23. *J Am Board Fam Pract.* 2004 May-Jun;17(3):212–9.
24. *JAMA.* 1997;277:32–7.
25. *Am Fam Physician.* 2005 Oct 1;72(7):1309–10.
26. *Sleep.* 2005 May 1;28(5):611–5.
27. *Ther Umsch.* 2000 Apr;57(4):241–5.
28. *J Clin Psychopharmacol.* 1996 Dec;16(6):428–36.
29. *Int J Biomed Sci.* 2005 Jun 15;1(1):33-45.
30. *Int J Biomed Sci.* 2006 Jun;2(2):143-59.
31. *Int J Biomed Sci.* 2006 Dec 15;2(4):375-94.
32. *Eur Respir J.* 2001 May;17(5):838–47.
33. *Planta Med.* 2001 Nov;67(8):695–9.
34. *Pharmacol Biochem Behav.* 1982 Jul;17(1):65–71.
35. *Planta Med.* 1985;2:144–8.
36   *ACP J Club.* 2004;141:A14–A16.
37. *Altern Med Rev.* 2004 Dec;9(4):438–41.
38. *Eur J Med Res.* 2002 Nov 25;7(11):480–6.
39. *CNS Spectr.* 2001 Oct;6(10):841–7.
40   *J Am Pharm Assoc* (Wash). 1999 Sep-Oct;39(5):688–96.
41. *Pharmacopsychiatry.* 1999;32:235–41.
42. *Pharmacol Biochem Behav.* 2004 May;78(1):57–64.
43. *Am Fam Physician.* 2003 Apr 15;67(8):1755–8.
44. *Arzneimittelforschung.* 1995;45:753–5.
45. *Anesth Analg.* 2004 Feb;98(2):353–8.
46. *Drug Metab Dispos.* 2004 Dec;32(12):1333–6.
47. *J Pharm Pharm Sci.* 2004 Aug 12;7(2):265–73.
48. *Phytother Res.* 2005 Sep;19(9):801–3.
49. *Altern Med Rev.* 1998 Aug;3(4):271–80.
50. *MMW Fortschr Med.* 2005 May 17;147 Spec No 2:7–11.
51. *Nutr Neurosci.* 2005 Apr;8(2):121–7.
52. *Phytomedicine.* 2006 15 Feb.
53. *Psychosom Med.* 2004 Jul-Aug;66(4):607–13.

Life Extension®
Diet Program

Nutrition and physical activity are critical components for life-long health. As committed as you are to your short-term weight loss goals, *Life Extension* is equally committed to providing the tools you need to help you optimize your success over the long term.

Life Extension recommends a program to include physical activity and a nutritional strategy that emphasizes complex carbohydrates and dietary fiber.

Fiber-rich Foods High in Complex Carbohydrates

What foods are rich in both dietary fiber and complex carbohydrates? For a start, consider whole grains like whole wheat, brown rice, wild rice, whole oats, buckwheat, barley, and other whole grains.

Other foods rich in fiber and complex carbohydrates are legumes like lentils and beans. Yams, sweet potatoes, squash, and plantains are also good sources of complex carbohydrates and dietary fiber. Of course, vegetables and whole fruits (not fruit juices, which are a concentrated source of fructose calories) are excellent sources of vitamins, minerals, and dietary fiber.

As a practical example, substituting whole wheat pasta instead of regular spaghetti is one of the easiest ways to boost your intake of complex carbohydrates and dietary fiber. Other easy choices, readily available at grocery stores and supermarkets, are yams or sweet potatoes. If whole grains or legumes won't be at the center of your meal, there are plenty of other choices for delectable dishes packed with dietary fiber and complex carbohydrates at dinner. Try brown rice pilaf, mashed cauliflower, spicy bean dip with sliced, raw veggies, or just toss some chickpeas or kidney beans into a green salad with a splash of extra virgin olive oil and fresh lemon juice.

Here are some recommendations to consider for optimal success along with this complex carbohydrate, fiber-rich diet:

- Drinking 8 glasses of water daily (about 64 ounces total) helps you stay hydrated and supports metabolic function, helping to process and excrete toxins from the body.

- Adequate protein in the form of fish, lean poultry, nonfat dairy and complemented proteins are needed daily, with the goal of reaching at least 60 grams total. Most Americans eat far too much protein than needed, often at the expense of their pocketbooks (because meat is expensive!) and to the strain of the kidneys and liver, both of which help process excess protein. Just 4–6 ounces of fish or poultry, a serving of non-fat dairy products such as 8 ounces of skim or soy milk, and fiber-rich, complex carbohydrates can be complemented with nuts and seeds to provide added protein and fiber. For example, whole grain bread and almond butter (or peanut butter) make a complete protein. Tofu and other soy foods are also good sources of plant protein as well.

- Remember the better ways to cook food: steam, bake, broil or poach, but avoid frying and grilling.

- Four to six servings of whole fruits and vegetables daily should be a part of your plan. Try to stay away from fruit juices and eat whole, fresh fruits and vegetables instead so you benefit from the fiber to assist in maintaining healthy blood glucose levels, delay hunger, and assist with digestion.

- Avoid fat-rich gravies, sauces, spreads and toppings unless they are low in fat, especially saturated fats. Use spices instead of fat to flavor food.

- Get your crock pot out and start experimenting with beans, lentils, and peas to make low-cost, easy, hearty and healthy soups your whole family can enjoy! Crock pot cooking is one of the easiest ways to make home-cooked, inexpensive meals.

- Potato chips, bakery muffins, bagels slathered in cream cheese, and corn crisps are a few examples of foods high in complex carbohydrates but also fiber-poor and fat-rich. These are not good food choices. Keep in mind that you can easily convert a low fat food rich in complex carbohydrate and fiber into a calorie surplus – for example, a simple baked potato is rich in complex carbohydrate and fiber, but slathered with butter or sour cream quickly becomes a calorie disaster. A better choice would be fiber-rich salsa with your potato.

- If you need to eat at a restaurant, make sensible food choices, emphasizing fiber-rich foods and minimizing fat-laden entrees. Ask for steamed vegetables with herbs, not sautéed vegetables in butter or oil.

- Ask your doctor if you can exercise. Increasing energy expenditure and maintaining lean muscle mass are always important ingredients to a healthy lifestyle. You will feel better physically and emotionally, with better energy and improved strength.

Menu Planning

Here is a range of serving values to help you get started on your weight-management program:

Whole grain bread, cereal, brown rice, whole grain pasta, and potatoes: 5–7 servings per day
1 serving = 1 slice of bread, 1 ounce dry cereal, ½ cup cooked cereal, ½ cup cooked brown rice, ½ cup cooked whole grain pasta, 1 small baked potato or ½ cup sweet potato.

Vegetables: 3–5 servings per day
1 serving = 1 cup raw leafy greens, ½ cup any other chopped raw or cooked vegetable; do not use vegetable juice.

Fruits: 2–4 servings per day
1 serving = 1 medium apple, banana, or orange; ½ cup chopped fruit or berries; do not use fruit juice.

Low Fat Milk, Yogurt (plain, not sweetened), and Cheese: 2–4 servings per day
1 serving = 1 cup milk or yogurt, 1 ½ ounces of natural cheese, 2 ounces of processed cheese.

Meat, Poultry, Fish, Dry Beans, Eggs, and Nuts: 2–3 servings a day
1 serving = 2–3 ounces of cooked lean meat, poultry, or fish; 1 egg; ½ cup cooked beans, 2 tablespoons peanut butter, nuts, or seeds.

Sample Meals:

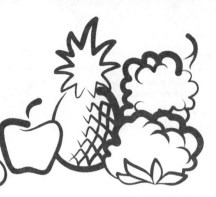

Day 1:

BREAKFAST
- 1 ounce of whole grain ready-to-eat cereal or ½ cup of oatmeal made from whole rolled oats
- ½ cup fresh fruit
- 1 - 8 ounce glass of skim milk or a 4 ounce serving of fat-free cottage cheese

SNACK
- 1 fruit, such as a medium banana

LUNCH
- Peanut butter sandwich made with 2 slices of whole grain bread
- ½ cup carrot sticks
- ½ cup blueberries
- 1 ½ ounces cheese

SNACK
- 15–20 almonds

DINNER
- 1 cup whole wheat pasta tossed with 2 tablespoons of toasted sesame seeds and 4 ounces of broiled salmon chunks, drizzled with low sodium soy sauce
- Salad, lightly dressed with lemon juice, vinegar and olive oil blend
- ½ cup zucchini and yellow squash medallions baked, steamed or broiled with herbs and onions
- ½ cup melon

Day 2:

BREAKFAST
- 1 slice of whole grain toast
- 1 egg
- ½ cup berries
- 1 cup nonfat plain yogurt

SNACK
- 1 fruit, such as a medium apple

LUNCH
- 1 cup split pea and lentil soup
- ½ cup whole grain cooked pasta
- 2 tablespoons tomato sauce or 1 sliced tomato
- ½ cup steamed or raw broccoli, can be tossed with pasta and tomato or tomato sauce

SNACK
- 2 tablespoons of walnuts

DINNER
- 4 ounces of lean meat, fish or poultry
- Salad, lightly dressed with lemon juice, vinegar and olive oil blend
- ½ cup baked sweet potato, no butter or dressing, just herbs to taste
- 1 - 8 ounce cup skim milk
- ½ cup fresh strawberries or melon

Day 3:

BREAKFAST
- 2 ounces of dry whole grain cereal
- 1 cup skim milk
- ½ cup sliced banana

SNACK
- 1 fruit, such as a medium orange

LUNCH
- 4 ounces grilled fish or 1 cup nonfat cottage cheese
- 1 slice whole grain toast
- 1 teaspoon fruit preserves
- 1 cup raw or steamed string beans

SNACK
- 2 tablespoons of sunflower seeds

DINNER
- 3 ounces of lean meat or poultry
- Salad, lightly dressed with lemon juice, vinegar and olive oil blend
- ½ cup potato crisps (thinly sliced potato brushed lightly with olive oil and herbs, baked)
- ½ cup fresh mango

Day 4:

BREAKFAST
- 1 cup cooked whole grain cereal
- 1 cup nonfat plain yogurt
- ½ cup berries

SNACK
- 1 fruit, such as ½ cup apricots

LUNCH
- 2 ounces cheese (melt into pasta)
- 1 cup whole grain pasta
- 1 cup broccoli (steamed or raw, mix in with pasta or on the side)
- ½ teaspoon olive oil (mixed into pasta), if needed

SNACK
- 15–20 almonds

DINNER
- 4 ounces of lean meat or poultry, or 4 ounces tofu
- ½ cup cooked greens (mustard, kale, etc.), seasoned with garlic or other herbs
- ½ cup brown rice
- ½ cup melon

Day 5:

BREAKFAST
- 2 slices of whole grain toast
- 1 egg
- 1 medium orange
- 1 ounce cheese

SNACK
- ½ cup berries

LUNCH
- ½ cup beans (cooked and seasoned with spice)
- 3 tablespoons hummus
- 1 cup carrots and cucumber slices to dip
- 1 - 8 ounce cup skim milk

SNACK
- 2 tablespoons of walnuts

DINNER
- 4 ounces of lean meat, fish, or poultry
- Spinach salad, lightly dressed with lemon juice, vinegar and olive oil blend
- ½ cup baked sweet potato, no butter or dressing, just herbs to taste
- ½ cup fresh papaya

Day 6:

BREAKFAST
- 1 ounce of whole grain ready-to-eat cereal or ½ cup of oatmeal made from whole rolled oats
- ½ cup fresh fruit
- 1 - 8 ounce glass of skim milk or a 4 ounce serving of fat-free cottage cheese

SNACK
- 1 fruit, such as a medium banana

LUNCH
- 4 ounces fish or chicken
- 1 cup whole grain pasta seasoned with 1 teaspoon olive oil, garlic and black pepper
- ½ cup spinach
- ½ cup berries
- 1 ounce part skim cheese

SNACK
- 15–20 cashews

DINNER
- 4 ounces lean meat or poultry seasoned to taste
- Salad, lightly dressed with lemon juice, vinegar and olive oil blend
- ½ cup zucchini and yellow squash medallions baked, steamed or broiled with herbs and onions
- 1 small baked potato, seasoned to taste with Butter Buds®
- ½ cup melon

Day 7:

BREAKFAST
- 1 slice of whole grain toast
- 1 egg
- ½ cup berries
- 1 cup nonfat plain yogurt

SNACK
- 1 fruit, such as a medium pear

LUNCH
- 1 cup minestrone soup
- 2 slices whole grain flatbread
- ½ cup steamed or raw broccoli, can be tossed with pasta and tomato or tomato sauce
- 1 - 8 ounce glass of skim milk or a 4 ounce serving of fat-free cottage cheese

SNACK
- 15–20 almonds

DINNER
- 4 ounces of lean meat, fish or poultry sautéed with garlic cloves, 1 cup red and green peppers
- Salad, lightly dressed with lemon juice, vinegar and olive oil blend
- ½ cup baked sweet potato, no butter or dressing, just herbs to taste
- 1 - 8 ounce cup skim milk
- ½ cup fresh fruit

If you have any questions on the scientific content of this book, please call a Life Extension Health Advisor at 1-866-820-8083.

You Can Do It!

You have made a life-altering decision! You're <u>not</u> going to tolerate unsightly **body fat** any longer. And, you're <u>not</u> going to feel chronically **tired** because of excess body weight.

Most importantly, you're <u>not</u> going to place yourself at greater risk of **cancer**, **heart attack**, **stroke**, **arthritis**, and **Alzheimer's disease** because you <u>store</u> too many fat pounds.

Having said that, let's examine what is causing **you** to be heavier than you'd like.

First of all, are you **sleeping** well? Sleep deprivation increases appetite and diabetes risk. We included a chapter on combating insomnia in this weight-loss program to make sure you start off on the right track.

Second, we want to remind everyone that humans have evolved to *efficiently* utilize ingested calories. This means people readily break down foods in the digestive tract, absorb the bulk of these calories into the bloodstream, and then **hoard** <u>excess</u> calories in the form of **body fat**.

As we age, the propensity to <u>accumulate</u> unwanted body fat increases for a variety of reasons. The purpose of the weight-loss protocols you have read is to address <u>multiple</u> obesity factors.

As you have learned, aging people often need to do <u>more</u> to achieve desired body weight than younger individuals. That's why we have worked around-the-clock to develop the most <u>comprehensive</u> weight-management program in medical history.

The data described in this book can enable you to identify what may be causing <u>you</u> to be overweight. Correcting these multiple, scientifically identified obesity factors provides a comprehensive strategy to shed those excess fat pounds.

Yours in health,
Steven V. Joyal, M.D. and William Faloon